Student Laboratory Manual for

Seidel's Guide to Physical Examination
An Interprofessional Approach

10th edition

Jane W. Ball, DrPH, RN, CPNP
Chief Nursing and Content Officer, Triaj, Inc
Havre de Grace, Maryland

**Joyce E. Dains, DRPH, JD, APRN,
FNP-BC, FNAP, FAANP, FAAN**
Professor and Chair, ad interim
Department of Nursing
Executive Director Advanced Practice
The University of Texas
M. D. Anderson Cancer Center
Houston, Texas

John A. Flynn, MD, MBA, MEd
Professor of Medicine
Department of Medicine
The University of Chicago
Chicago, Illinois

Barry S. Solomon, MD, MPH
Professor of Pediatrics
Chief, Division of General Pediatrics
Assistant Dean for Medical Student Affairs
The Johns Hopkins University
School of Medicine
Baltimore, Maryland

Rosalyn W. Stewart, MD, MS, MBA
Professor of Medicine and Pediatrics
The Johns Hopkins University
School of Medicine
Baltimore, Maryland

Student Laboratory Manual prepared by:
Frances D. Monahan, PhD, RN, ANEF
Nursing Education Consultant
Vero Beach, Florida

ELSEVIER

Elsevier
3251 Riverport Lane
St. Louis, Missouri 63043

STUDENT LABORATORY MANUAL FOR SEIDEL'S GUIDE TO
PHYSICAL EXAMINATION: AN INTERPROFESSIONAL APPROACH, TENTH EDITION

ISBN: 978-0-323-77604-2

Executive Content Strategist: Lee Henderson
Senior Content Development Manager: Luke Held
Publishing Services Manager: Sheeren Jameel
Project Manager: Aparna Venkatachalam

Printed in India

Last digit is the print number: 9 8 7 6 5 4 3 2 1

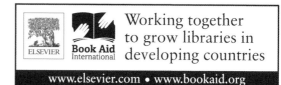

Preface

This *Student Laboratory Manual for Mosby's Guide to Physical Examination: An Interprofessional Approach,* 10th edition, has been designed to help you achieve the goals associated with learning to interview patients for a health history and to perform physical examinations. Each chapter corresponds to one in the textbook, with the same title and chapter number. The correct answers to the questions are listed in the back of the Student *Laboratory Manual* so that you can evaluate your comprehension of the material.

Each chapter begins with a list of Learning Objectives for use in assessing your comprehension of the material. A variety of exercises in each chapter help you practice and confirm your understanding of the concepts, key terms, and techniques of examination. These exercises include the following:

- **Terminology Review:** Fill-in-the-blank exercises with key terms and definitions help you master the language of health assessment and physical examination.

- **Concepts Application:** Exercises will help you evaluate and assess examination findings to interpret the results and recognize normal and abnormal outcomes.

- **Case Study:** Case Studies give you the opportunity to apply data evaluation skills in a clinical setting. Additional information or data needed to further determine a diagnosis or course of action may be called for, and you will have the opportunity to suggest further examination.

- **Clinical Reasoning:** Problems are posed to give you practice in analyzing patient information and managing interactions with patients, with additional questions focused on patient safety.

- **Content Review Questions:** Multiple-choice, fill-in-the-blank, and matching questions will help you review the primary concepts and terminology related to the content. Anatomic drawings to be labeled will challenge you to apply knowledge associated with the relevant body systems.

It is my hope that the Student *Laboratory Manual* will be helpful to you in your study of physical examination.

Frances D. Monahan, PhD, RN, ANEF

Contents

1 Cultural Competency

After studying Chapter 1 in the textbook and completing this section of the laboratory manual, students should be able to:
1. Define cultural competence, cultural humility, and cultural awareness.
2. Examine differences and similarities between ethnic and physical characteristics.
3. Analyze the impact of culture on illness, health beliefs, and practices.
4. Examine modes of communication that explore a patient's culture.
5. Discuss healthcare delivery for transgender and gender-diverse (TGD) people

TERMINOLOGY REVIEW

Check your understanding of terminology related to cultural competency. Using the space provided, write the word or phrase from the list next to the appropriate descriptor.

Culture
Cultural awareness
Cultural desire
Cultural humility

Cultural knowledge
Culturally competent care
Cultural skill
Genomics
Precision Medicine
Stereotype

1. _____: the process of seeking and obtaining a sound educational base about culturally and ethnically diverse groups.

2. _____: the ability to recognize one's limitations in knowledge and cultural perspective.

3. _____: study of multiple genes and their interactions with environmental determinants, in predicting disease susceptibility and response to medical treatment.

4. _____: reflection of the whole spectrum of human behavior, including ideas and attitudes.

5. _____: motivation of a healthcare professional to "want to" engage in the process of becoming culturally competent.

6. _____: sensitivity to the patient's heritage, sexual orientation, socioeconomic situation, ethnicity, and cultural background.

7. _____: the deliberate self-examination of one's biases, stereotypes, prejudices, and assumptions about cultures that are different from one's own.

8. _____: an inflexible generalization about a group.

9. _____: an approach to the prevention and treatment of disease that takes into account an individual's genetic profile, environment, and lifestyle.

10. _____: the ability to collect culturally relevant data regarding the patient's presenting problem.

1

Clinical Case Study

A 52-year-old Chinese woman presents to your practice with a complaint of burning pain in the abdomen that occurs 3–4 times per week. She speaks very little English and arrives without her family to assist with communication.

1. What is your first consideration as you prepare for the assessment of this patient?

2. What questions could you ask that explore the patient's culture?

3. What questions could you ask to find out about any culturally traditional treatment(s) she has already tried?

4. What might the patient have tried as a self-treatment for her abdominal pain if she practices the hot and cold belief system?

Concepts Application

When working with sexual or gender minorities (SGM), healthcare providers are responsible for providing a welcoming and safe environment, gathering a history with sensitivity and compassion, and performing a physical examination using a "gender-affirming" approach. Fulfilling these responsibilities begins with understanding gender, transgender, and sexuality terminology. Check your understanding of these terms by writing the appropriate term in the box to the left of its definition.

Terms:

Gender-diverse

Gender/gender identity

Nonbinary

Sex

Sexual orientation

Transgender

Term	Definition
	Person whose gender identity differs from that sex assigned at birth but may be more complex or fluid. It can encompass individuals who identify as non-binary, genderqueer, gender fluid, and a host of other descriptors.
	A person's sexual, romantic, emotional, and physical attraction toward other people.
	Person whose gender identity differs from sex assigned at birth.
	A person's internal sense of self and how they fit into the world from the perspective of gender.
	Not identifying as exclusively male or female within the traditional gender binary of Western European-based culture.
Sex	Sex assigned at birth, historically based on a cursory visualization of external genitalia.

Clinical Reasoning Case Study 1

A 45-year-old Hispanic transgender man presents to your office with a complaint of sore throat, fever, and fatigue. You make the diagnosis of infectious mononucleosis and recommend that he take 2 weeks off from work.

1. How do you define a transgender man?

2. Because the patient is Hispanic, his belief system may include the need for a balance between hot and cold. What hot and cold remedies might he have tried already to self-treat his condition?

Clinical Reasoning Case Study 2

You are caring for a minority patient who has a chronic illness requiring dietary teaching and education about medications. Listed below are areas for cultural assessment. For each area, list at least one question you could ask as part of a cultural assessment to better prepare for this patient's care.

1. Health beliefs and practices

2. Religious and ritual influences

3. Dietary practices

4. Family relationships and relational orientation

Self Reflection

Reflect on your care of patients of different cultures. What were your strengths in providing culturally competent care? What barriers to providing culturally competent care did you encounter? How did you manage your differences?

CONTENT REVIEW QUESTIONS

Multiple Choice

Circle the best answer for each of the following questions.

1. Which phrase refers to healthcare that incorporates information about an individual's genes, proteins, and environment into the prevention, diagnosis, and treatment of disease?
   a. Culturally skilled medicine
   b. Culturally aware medicine
   c. Genomic medicine
   d. Personalized medicine

2. The balance of hot and cold and its relationship to wellness is a belief system that
   a. is reductionist in its focus on a very narrow, specific cause and effect of illness.
   b. is encountered only in populations from underdeveloped nations.
   c. has led to poor sanitization practices in many areas of the world.
   d. is held by members of many cultures, including Arab, Asian, Filipino, and Hispanic.

3. Developing a knowledge base about cultural groups allows the practitioner to
   a. predict with complete accuracy the behavior and attitude of the patient.
   b. use stereotypic judgments to anticipate the patient's need for instruction and support.
   c. understand the behaviors, practices, and problems observed.
   d. change the behavior or practices of the patient to conform to healthcare practice.

4. Which of the following is an example of a cultural characteristic?
   a. Skin color
   b. Intelligence
   c. Skull size
   d. Shared belief

5. An integral part of the overall effort to respond adequately to a person in need is
   a. cultural awareness.
   b. ethnocentric bias.
   c. political correctness.
   d. racial alertness.

6. A young mother brings her infant to the clinic because the infant "is irritable, very fussy, and not eating." Which of the following questions asked by an examiner demonstrates cultural awareness?
   a. "When did the symptoms begin?"
   b. "What do you think is causing this illness?"
   c. "Has your child been exposed to any sick children recently?"
   d. "What have you already done at home to manage your child's illness?"

7. Which is the best description of a culturally competent healthcare provider?
   a. A healthcare provider who is genuinely curious about the beliefs and values of patients from varied backgrounds.
   b. A healthcare provider who adapts to the unique needs of patients with backgrounds and beliefs that differ from his or her own.
   c. A healthcare provider who appreciates diversity and is aware of health disparities.
   d. A healthcare provider who avoids stereotyping and treats all patients with respect.

8. A common mistake made by healthcare professionals is to
   a. acknowledge the practice of folk or herbal remedies.
   b. adapt healthcare concepts to meet the needs of individuals of other cultures.
   c. stereotype individuals based on color or ethnic group.
   d. carefully assess the understanding and beliefs of culturally diverse individuals.

9. All of the following are cultural considerations that affect healthcare *except*
   a. eye color, temperature, and visual acuity.
   b. social class, age, and gender.
   c. ethnic traditions, level of education, and family relationships.
   d. religious beliefs, dietary habits, and mode of communication.

10. Which of the following is an example of a physical, as opposed to a cultural, characteristic?
    a. Language
    b. Hair style
    c. Skin color
    d. Religious affiliation

11. Despite repeated instruction over a period of 3 years, the mother of three young children has still not had her children immunized. Which of the following questions would help the healthcare provider understand this situation?
    a. "When are you going to get your children immunized?"
    b. "What are your beliefs about immunizations?"
    c. "We have asked you to get your children immunized. Why has this not been done?"
    d. "Don't you understand that your children may get ill without immunizations?"

12. Which mode of communication may be offensive to a patient whose cultural perspective differs from that of the practitioner?
    a. Speaking in modulated tones
    b. Allowing quiet time for reflection during an interview
    c. Using reflection to repeat and clarify the information
    d. Maintaining firm and direct eye contact

13. Which of the following statements is an accurate interpretation of the concept of balancing hot and cold?
    a. Treatment to restore hot and cold balance requires the use of opposites.
    b. The recommended treatment for a "cold" condition is to serve cold foods.
    c. The recommended treatment for a "hot" condition is hot foods and cold medications.
    d. Ailments and treatments considered "hot" or "cold" are related to the effect of body temperature.

14. Which is an example of social transition from living aligned with one's sex assigned at birth to living aligned with one's gender identity?
    a. Having a driver's license altered
    b. Changing appearance by wearing a wig
    c. Engaging in speech therapy
    d. Taking hormones

2 The History and Interviewing Process

After studying Chapter 2 in the textbook and completing this section of the laboratory manual, students should be able to:
1. Classify aspects of communication that affect the interview process.
2. Obtain a comprehensive health history.
3. Apply the elements of a clinical presentation to a health history.
4. Organize data according to a clinical history outline.
5. Differentiate between the history and interviewing process used for an adult patient with the process used for patients of special populations, such as patients with disabilities, pregnant patients, and frail patients.

TERMINOLOGY REVIEW

Check your understanding of terminology related to the history and interviewing process. Using the space provided, write the word or phrase from the list next to the appropriate descriptor.

CAGE

Chief concern (CC)

Family history (FH)

Functional assessment

History of present illness (HPI)

Intimate partner violence (IPV)

Past medical history (PMH)

Personal and social history (SH)

Review of systems (ROS)

Symptom analysis

1. _____: a range of abusive behaviors perpetrated by someone who is or was involved in an intimate relationship with the victim.

2. _____: questions specifying the onset, location, duration, intensity, characteristics, and aggravating and alleviating factors.

3. _____: questionnaire for discussing the use of alcohol, which includes cutting down, annoyance by criticism, guilty, and eye openers.

4. _____: blood relatives in the immediate or extended family with illnesses that have features similar to the patient's concern.

5. _____: a brief statement of the reason the patient is seeking care.

6. _____: work, marriage, sexual, and spiritual experiences; the patient's use of alcohol, tobacco, and drugs.

7. _____: questions concerning the ability to take care of one's daily needs that are part of the review of systems.

8. _____: the patient's state of overall health before the present problem.

9. _____: a step-by-step evaluation of the circumstances that surround the primary reason for the patient's visit.

10. _____: the presence or absence of health-related issues in each body system.

Clinical Case Study

A 25-year-old woman presents to your office with fatigue. She is a college graduate, but currently working as a waitress because she has not been able to secure a job in her field.

1. What is this patient's chief complaint?

2. What questions would you ask to complete the HPI?

3. What is your goal when you do the ROS?

4. What systems would you ask questions about during the ROS?

Concepts Application

Listed below are patient behaviors/issues that can create tension for the examiner. For each patient behavior/issue listed, provide a behavior by the examiner that could help decrease the tension. (Write your answers in the space provided in the right-hand column.)

Patient Behavior/Issue	Examiner Behavior to Decrease Tension
Seduction	
Depression	
Anxiety	
Excessive flattery	
Financial concerns	
Silence	

Clinical Reasoning Case Study 1

A 35-year-old man presents to your office with a complaint of left foot pain. He describes this as a severe burning pain on the outside edge of the heel of his left foot. The pain is worse in the morning and when he walks barefoot. The pain improves when he applies ice to his foot. In addition, the patient states, "I have been using Tylenol one or two times per day." The pain started 2 weeks ago after the patient was walking on the beach. The pain lasts for 2 to 3 hours in the morning and then seems to subside after he is up and walking for a while.

1. Based on the information in this case study, identify each of the following characteristics of the patient's pain using the mnemonic device "OLDCARTS."

   Onset:

   Location:

   Duration:

   Characteristics:

   Aggravating factors:

   Relieving factors:

   Timing:

   Severity:

7

A 52-year-old woman presents to your office with sudden burning and stabbing pain in the left orbit. She says her pain is severe, and she is outwardly agitated. She experienced similar pain the day before at about the same time. She denies associated signs or symptoms of nausea or vomiting, aura, new medications, and excessive alcohol use. She reports a 24-year pack history for smoking and says she has high stress on her job, does daily exercise, and follows a prudent diet. Her past history is unremarkable with the exception of "spells" of headaches similar to this from time to time. According to the patient, these symptoms occur without warning and resolve after a few hours but usually return the next day. This may go on for a week or more before the symptoms stop until the next episode begins.

1. What components of a health history are present in this case study?

2. What component(s) should have been added to the health history?

3. What components are only partially complete?

Patient Safety Consideration

When might you consider breaking the confidentiality of patient–healthcare provider communication?

CONTENT REVIEW QUESTIONS

Multiple Choice

Circle the best answer for each of the following questions.

1. Which of the following actions will best facilitate the interview when obtaining a history from a deaf patient who can read lips?
   a. Speaking loudly
   b. Using gestures
   c. Speaking slowly
   d. Sitting to the side of the patient

2. Approximately what percentage of patients interviewed have a sexual orientation other than heterosexual?
   a. 2%
   b. 5%
   c. 10%
   d. 20%

3. During a history, the patient indicates that he has an uncle and a brother with sickle cell disease. Which of the following is an appropriate method by which to document this information?
   a. Document this as chief complaint.
   b. Include it in the family history.
   c. Include this in the past medical history.
   d. Incorporate this information in the social history.

4. Which approach is recommended at the onset of an interview?
   a. Ask questions in a structured manner.
   b. Introduce yourself, giving details of your background and qualifications.
   c. Be open-ended, letting the patient explain the problem or reason for the visit.
   d. Explain the need for family history and past medical history to determine the underlying problem.

5. Which of the following questions would be the most likely to elicit an inaccurate patient response?
   a. "Where do you feel the pain?"
   b. "How does this situation make you feel?"
   c. "What happened after you noticed your injury?"
   d. "That was a horrible experience, wasn't it?"

6. Repeating a patient's answer is an attempt to
   a. confirm an accurate understanding.
   b. discourage patient anger or hostility.
   c. teach the patient new medical terms.
   d. allow the patient to change his or her response.

7. Which of the following is unique to a pediatric history?
   a. Family history
   b. Developmental history
   c. Social history
   d. Past medical history

8. When interviewing an adolescent who is reluctant to talk during an interview, it is best to
   a. tell the patient you must have honest answers to your questions.
   b. reassure the patient that information discussed is confidential.
   c. inform the patient that adolescents often have trouble expressing their feelings.
   d. obtain the history from a parent or other family member.

9. During an interview, your patient admits to feeling worthless and having a sleep disturbance for the past 3 weeks. These are clues that warrant the exploration of
   a. risk for suicide.
   b. split personality.
   c. cognitive function.
   d. functional assessment.

10. Which finding indicates a positive Partner Violence Screen (PVS)?
    a. A positive response to any one question
    b. A score of 6 or higher
    c. Presence of unexplained body bruising
    d. History of 3 or more healthcare encounters for accidental injuries within a year

11. Which questionnaire developed to screen for drug and alcohol use is recommended for adolescent patients?
    a. AUDIT-C
    b. CAGE
    c. CRAFFT
    d. TACE

12. A 26-year-old homosexual man, is having a health history taken. Which question regarding sexual activity would most likely *hamper* trust between him and the interviewer?
    a. "Are you married, or do you have a girlfriend?"
    b. "Tell me about your living situation."
    c. "Are you sexually active?"
    d. "Are your partners men, women, or both?"

13. A conversation with a parent concerning a 5-year-old child
    a. violates the child's need for privacy.
    b. is inappropriate because the child is able to talk with you.
    c. provides significant information about family dynamics.
    d. causes distrust in the child toward the examiner.

14. Long periods of silence during an interview may indicate
    a. a need for the healthcare provider to increase the pace of the interview.
    b. an inability of the patient to communicate.
    c. time needed to gain courage to discuss a painful topic.
    d. a need to terminate the interview because of the patient's inability to pay attention.

15. When questioning a patient regarding a sensitive issue, such as drug use, it is best to
    a. begin by describing to the patient the relationship of the issue to health.
    b. be direct, firm, and to the point.
    c. explain that the information will be shared only with healthcare workers.
    d. apologize to the patient for asking personal questions.

16. Direct questions are designed to
    a. attack sensitive material head on.
    b. demonstrate to the patient who is in charge of the interview process.
    c. ensure confidentiality.
    d. obtain or clarify specific details about an answer.

17. Interviewers should identify and assess their own feelings, such as hostility and prejudice, in order to
    a. avoid inappropriate behavior.
    b. explain their biases to patients.
    c. express their idiosyncrasies.
    d. reduce communication barriers.

18. During an interview, a patient describes abdominal pain that often awakens him at night. Which of the following responses by the interviewer would facilitate the interviewing process?
    a. "Constipation can cause abdominal pain."
    b. "Do you need a sleeping medication?"
    c. "Pain is always worse at night, isn't it?"
    d. "Tell me what you mean by *often.*"

9

19. When taking a patient's history, you are asked questions about your personal life. What is the best response to facilitate the interviewing process?
    a. Answer briefly and then refocus to the patient's history.
    b. Give as much detail as possible about the asked information.
    c. Ignore the question and continue with the patient's history.
    d. Tell the patient that it is inappropriate to answer personal questions.

20. During an interview, the patient describes problems associated with an illness and begins to cry. The best action in this situation is to
    a. stop the interview and reschedule for another time.
    b. allow the patient to cry and then resume when the patient is ready.
    c. change the topic to something less upsetting.
    d. continue the interview while the patient cries in order to get through it quickly.

3 Examination Techniques and Equipment

After studying Chapter 3 in the textbook and completing this section of the laboratory manual, students should be able to:
1. Apply standard precautions for infection control to the examination process.
2. Correctly obtain baseline data (vital signs, height, and weight).
3. Describe the meaning of base line data findings.
4. Differentiate various types of equipment used for physical examination.
5. Describe the purpose of various types of equipment used for physical examination.
6. Demonstrate the correct use of various types of equipment used for physical examination.
7. Identify various techniques applied during a physical examination.
8. Describe the purpose of various techniques used during a physical examination.
9. Demonstrate correct application of the various techniques used during physical examination.

TERMINOLOGY REVIEW

Check your understanding of terminology related to examination techniques and equipment. Using the space provided, write the word or phrase from the list next to the appropriate descriptor.

Amsler grid
Aperture setting
Bell of stethoscope
Diaphragm of stethoscope
Doppler
Goniometer
Ophthalmoscope

Otoscope
Percussion
Snellen chart
Stadiometer
Transilluminator
Tuning fork
Tympanometer
Wood's lamp

1. _____: examination technique that involves striking one object against another to produce vibration and subsequent sound waves.

2. _____: the part of the stethoscope that detects low-frequency sounds.

3. _____: an instrument used to determine the degree of flexion or extension of a joint.

4. _____: a device used to screen patients at risk for macular degeneration.

5. _____: an instrument used for screening tests for auditory function and for vibratory sensation.

6. _____: device used to measure the height of persons able to stand erect without support.

7. _____: an instrument that allows the examiner to evaluate the internal eye structures.

8. _____: a function that adjusts or changes light variations of an ophthalmoscope for examination.

9. _____: an instrument that allows the examiner to evaluate the external auditory canal and the tympanic membrane.

10. _____: an instrument that differentiates tissue, fluid, and air within a body cavity.

11. _____: technology that detects blood flow.

12. _____: an instrument used to assess function of the middle ear.

13. _____: the part of the stethoscope that detects high-pitched sounds.

14. _____: a tool used to test visual acuity for literate English-speaking patients.

15. _____: a black light used to detect fungi on skin lesions.

APPLICATION TO CLINICAL PRACTICE

Clinical Concepts Application 1

For each description listed below, provide the name of the examination technique or equipment described. (Write your answers in the space provided in the right-hand column.)

Description	Examination Technique or Equipment
Gathering information through touch	
Used to assess for macular degeneration	
Measures percentage of hemoglobin saturated with oxygen	
Source of light with a narrow beam	
Used to test deep tendon reflexes	
Used to visualize turbinates	
Assesses near vision	
Tests for loss of skin protective sensation	
Larger field of view in eye examination	

Clinical Concepts Application 2

Complete the following table by providing the expected examination findings. (Write your answers in the space provided in the right-hand column.)

Area Percussed	Percussion Tone Expected
Stomach	
Sternum	
Lung of patient with emphysema	
Liver	
Lung of patient with pneumonia	
Lung of normal patient	
Abdomen with large tumor	

Clinical Reasoning Case Study 1

1. A 72 year old woman is brought to the clinic by her daughter. She has an abdominal fistula that is draining foul, purulent fluid. She also has bowel and urinary incontinence. What infection control measures should be implemented?

Clinical Reasoning Case Study 2

A patient with a spinal cord injury at T5 requires a pelvic examination. On insertion of the vaginal speculum, the patient begins to sweat; her skin becomes blotchy; and she complains of nausea.

a. What is your immediate response?

b. Why?

Patient Safety Consideration

Why is it important for you, as the person performing physical assessments, to know your own strength?

CONTENT REVIEW QUESTIONS

Multiple Choice

Circle the best answer for each of the following questions.

1. Which of the following are the infection control guidelines currently recommended by the Centers for Disease Control and Prevention (CDC) for the care of all patients?
   a. Universal precautions
   b. Body substance isolation
   c. Standard precautions
   d. Illness-based precautions

2. A patient states that even after he urinates he doesn't feel like his bladder is really empty. Which instrument can be used to determine if his bladder incompletely empties?
   a. Calipers
   b. Tape measure
   c. Tympanometer
   d. Portable ultrasound unit

3. How does infection control practice in an outpatient setting such as a clinic compare with that in the acute-care setting?
   a. Transmission-based precautions are not used in an outpatient setting.
   b. Infection control is limited to protecting healthcare providers in the outpatient setting.
   c. The spread of infection to other patients is not a concern in the outpatient setting.
   d. Infection control practice is the same in acute and outpatient settings.

4. For which purpose is transillumination an appropriate examination technique?
   a. Assessment of vesicles on the skin
   b. Detection of fluid within the sinuses
   c. Measurement of bone density in the skull
   d. Determination of a mass in the liver

5. Which of the following instruments is used in conjunction with a simple nasal speculum to visualize the lower and middle turbinates of the nose?
   a. Otoscope
   b. Penlight
   c. Ophthalmoscope
   d. Goniometer

6. On first meeting, the examiner notices that the patient has an obvious odor. Which examination technique is the examiner using in this scenario?
   a. Inspection
   b. Palpation
   c. Percussion
   d. Auscultation

7. Focused visual attention obtains data from
   a. inspection.
   b. palpation.
   c. percussion.
   d. auscultation.

8. Which technique is applied throughout the entire examination and interview process?
   a. Inspection
   b. Palpation
   c. Percussion
   d. Auscultation

9. As a component of palpation, which surface is most sensitive to vibration?
   a. Fingertips
   b. Heel of the hand
   c. Dorsal surface of the hand
   d. Ulnar surface of the hand

10. The term *intensity*, when used in relation to percussion tones, refers to
    a. the loudness of the tone.
    b. the location of the tone.
    c. the musical quality of the tone.
    d. the length of duration the tone is heard.

11. Indirect finger percussion involves striking the middle finger of the nondominant hand with
    a. the fist.
    b. the percussion hammer.
    c. the tip of the middle finger of the dominant hand.
    d. the edge of the stethoscope disk.

12. A patient has a urinary tract infection. The examiner wishes to assess tenderness over the kidney. Which examination technique is appropriate?
    a. Light finger palpation over the kidney
    b. Firm fist percussion over the kidney
    c. Deep abdominal palpation of the kidney
    d. Auscultation for kidney bruit

13. The examiner has detected a superficial mass in the skin. What part of the hand is best to use to palpate this mass?
    a. Fingertips and fingers
    b. Heel of the hand
    c. Dorsal surface of the hand
    d. Ulnar surface of the hand

14. Ideally, auscultation should be carried out last, *except* when examining the
    a. lungs.
    b. heart.
    c. abdomen.
    d. kidney.

15. Which of the following techniques is *incorrect* and affects the accuracy of auscultation?
    a. Placing the stethoscope firmly on the surface to be auscultated
    b. Auscultating through clothing
    c. Isolating one sound at a time during auscultation
    d. Listening for sound characteristics

16. When measuring the length of an infant, the measurement should extend from the
    a. forehead to feet.
    b. top of head to heel in a prone position.
    c. head to toes in an upright position.
    d. crown to heel in a supine position.

17. The tubing of a stethoscope should be less than 18 inches long to prevent
    a. transmission of external noise.
    b. tangling of the tubing in the examiner's clothing.
    c. distortion of sounds during auscultation.
    d. magnification of the transmitted sounds.

18. Which of the following is true regarding the correct use of a stethoscope?
    a. The bell is pressed lightly against the skin to detect low-frequency sounds.
    b. The bell is pressed firmly against the skin to hear low-frequency sounds.
    c. The diaphragm is pressed firmly against the skin to hear low-frequency sounds.
    d. The diaphragm is pressed lightly against the skin to hear high-frequency sounds.

19. The examiner must be sure that the earpieces of the stethoscope are placed so that the alignment fits the contour of the ear canal. In which direction should they be placed?
    a. Pointing upward
    b. Pointing downward
    c. Pointing forward
    d. Pointing backward

20. In which of the following situations is use of a Doppler indicated?
    a. Measurement of body temperature in a hypothermic patient
    b. Auscultation of the abdomen in a patient with hypoactive or absent bowel sounds
    c. Measurement of blood pressure in a patient with a loud systolic sound
    d. Auscultation of a nonpalpable pulse in a patient with peripheral vascular disease

21. While performing an internal eye examination, the examiner observes a fundal lesion. What feature on the ophthalmoscope permits the examiner to estimate the size and location of the lesion?
    a. Grid aperture
    b. Slit aperture
    c. Red-free aperture
    d. Small aperture

22. An ophthalmoscope has positive and negative magnification in order to
    a. compensate for myopia or hyperopia in the examiner's or the patient's eyes.
    b. allow for magnification of both the anterior eye and the posterior eye.
    c. compensate for the degree of dilation of the patient's pupils.
    d. allow for visualization of the eye in patients with normal vision and in those with glaucoma.

23. In which of the following situations is the use of the pneumatic attachment of an otoscope indicated?
    a. Removal of excessive earwax from an adult or child
    b. Inflation of the ear canal for improved viewing in an adult with a collapsed canal
    c. Assessment of the fluctuating capacity of a child's tympanic membrane
    d. Evaluation of the cone of light reflex in an adult or child

24. The difference between a tuning fork for auditory screening and one for vibratory sensation is
    a. the sound frequency generated.
    b. the length of the tuning forks.
    c. the strike force needed on the forks.
    d. the auditory screening fork is electric; the vibratory fork is not.

25. Very young children may feel threatened by the use of a reflex hammer during examination. What could the examiner use in place of a reflex hammer that would be less threatening?
    a. Tuning fork
    b. Tongue blade
    c. End of a stethoscope
    d. Examiner's finger

26. According to the Centers for Disease Control and Prevention, the healthcare provider should apply infection control measures when caring for which group of patients?
    a. Patients with known infectious diseases
    b. Patients with possible infectious diseases
    c. Patients who appear ill
    d. All patients regardless of their infectious status

Taking the Next Steps: Critical Reasoning

LEARNING OBJECTIVES

After studying Chapter 4 in the textbook and completing this section of the laboratory manual, students should be able to:
1. Recognize ethical considerations in critical reasoning.
2. Discuss the process of data analysis.
3. Describe barriers to clinical reasoning in reaching diagnostic conclusions.
4. Identify terms associated with data analysis and problem identification.
5. Discuss the role of additional testing in the clinical examination process.
6. Describe what is meant by a patient management plan and explain where it fits with clinical reasoning and clinical examination.

TERMINOLOGY REVIEW

Check your understanding of terminology related to clinical reasoning. Using the space provided, write the word or phrase from the list next to the appropriate descriptor.

Autonomy
Bayes formula
Behavior change
Clinical reasoning
Evidence-based practice (EBP)
False negative
False positive
Negative predictive value

Nonmaleficence
Occam's razor
Positive predictive value
Sensitivity
Specificity
True negative
True positive

1. _____: an observation made that suggests a condition is not present when it actually is present.

2. _____: process of merging knowledge of the patient from interview and physical assessment, clinical experience, and current best evidence to determine patient care.

3. _____: the proportion of persons with an expected observation who ultimately prove not to have the expected condition.

4. _____: the ability of an observation to identify correctly those who have a disease.

5. _____: the likelihood of a diagnosis being related to the findings depends on the probability of those findings being associated with that diagnosis.

6. _____: an expected observation that is not found when the disease characterized by that observation is not present.

7. _____: a system that incorporates the best available scientific evidence to clinical decision-making in the care of the individual patient.

8. _____: a process involving progress through a series of stages.

9. _____: an expected observation that is found when the disease characterized by that observation is present.

10. _____: a principle stating that all findings should be unified into one diagnosis; this is not always true.

11. _____: the ability of an observation to identify correctly those who do not have the disease.

12. _____: an observation made that suggests a condition is present when it is not.

13. _____: the proportion of persons with an observation characteristic of a disease who actually have it.

14. _____: self determination; the right to choose between alternatives.

15. _____: do no harm to the patient.

APPLICATION TO CLINICAL PRACTICE

Concepts Application

Complete the following table by identifying the body systems that might be involved with each of the symptoms listed in the left-hand column below. Choose body systems from the following list. All symptoms have more than one possible body system involvement, and body systems can be used more than once.

Auditory   Musculoskeletal
Cardiovascular   Neurologic
Gastrointestinal   Respiratory
Integumentary   Visual

Symptoms	Body Systems that Might Be Involved
Chest pain	
Headaches	
Abdominal pain	
Pain in the legs	

Matching

Match each concept or method with the best example of its application.

Concept or Method	Example of Application
_____ 1. Recognizing patterns	a. Always consider potential harm as well as benefit.
_____ 2. Sampling the universe	b. If it looks like a cat; acts like a cat; it must be a cat.
_____ 3. Using algorithms	c. Including everything precludes missing anything.
_____ 4. Guidelines to decision-making	d. Rigidly defined thought process precludes error.

Chapter **4** **Taking the Next Steps: Critical Reasoning**

Matching

Match each concept with the scenario in which the term is applied. Use each concept only once.

Scenario	Concept
_____ 1. The examiner notes a positive Chvostek sign in the absence of hypocalcemia.	a. Bayes formula
_____ 2. The patient does not demonstrate tenderness at the McBurney point and does not have appendicitis.	b. False negative
	c. False positive
_____ 3. A numeric value is assigned, predicting the probability that a patient with negative findings does not have a given illness.	d. Negative predictive value
_____ 4. A diagnosis of hepatitis B infection is made based on the patient's symptoms and the population of intravenous drug abusers, of which he is part.	e. Positive predictive value
_____ 5. A patient with cholecystitis has a positive Murphy sign.	f. True positive
_____ 6. The examiner notes normal findings in a patient with prostate cancer.	g. True negative
_____ 7. With acute myocardial infarction, 90% of patients demonstrate diaphoresis.	

Concepts Application

Complete the following table by listing possible problems associated with the examination data provided.

Examination Data	Possible Problems
A 54-year-old woman with jaundice, abdominal pain, nausea, and weight loss. Has pain with abdominal palpation; positive bowel sounds. Liver slightly enlarged; admits to alcohol use.	
A 66-year-old man with a chief complaint of breathing difficulty. Has increased respiratory rate, low-grade fever, rales, productive cough; increased tactile fremitus bilaterally.	
A 13-week-old infant girl with fever, irritability, poor eating. Infant is dehydrated and has a temperature of 103.7° F; soft abdomen.	
A 19-year-old female college student with a chief complaint of pain when urinating. Describes frequency and urgency. Patient has temperature of 100.4° F; has constant pain in pelvic area; positive pain with fist percussion over left flank.	

CONTENT REVIEW QUESTIONS

Multiple Choice

Circle the best answer for each of the following questions.

1. What is the first step in clinical reasoning?
   a. Assessing the value and significance of information obtained from the patient
   b. Assigning a priority to the patient's symptoms
   c. Matching diagnostic test findings with patient history and physical examination data
   d. Combining objective and subjective data into an initial hypothesis

2. What is the foundation of clinical reasoning?
   a. Shared decision-making
   b. Evidence-based practice
   c. Problem list
   d. Examiner's hypothesis

3. After an examiner has identified and confirmed a problem, the next step is to
   a. assess the data collected.
   b. formulate a clinical opinion.
   c. conduct further assessment.
   d. determine the management plan.

4. What does Bayes Theorem describe?
   a. the risk of error in decision-making
   b. the probability of an observation being valid
   c. the likelihood of your diagnosis being related to your findings
   d. the prevalence of a particular diagnosis in a given community

5. Unless a life-threatening situation exists, the best guide to determining the priority for the patient's condition should be based on
   a. intuition.
   b. probability and utility.
   c. the use of algorithms.
   d. the examiner's initial favorite hypothesis.

6. Each of the following could become a barrier to the clinical reasoning process, *except* for the examiner's
   a. feelings.
   b. attitudes.
   c. values.
   d. objectivity.

7. Which statement best characterizes a belief that supports a sound decision-making process?
   a. The underlying problem is always related to the chief complaint.
   b. Rare problems tend to have unusual presentations.
   c. Common problems occur commonly, and rare ones occur rarely.
   d. A diagnosis should be made quickly to enhance patient confidence.

8. Laboratory tests should be used to
   a. confirm a presumed diagnosis.
   b. develop a list of potential problems.
   c. rule out all possible causes of symptoms and clinical findings.
   d. assist the examiner only when the data do not point to a specific problem.

9. A 62-year-old patient has been diagnosed with alcohol addiction. After discussing his situation, he tells you that he is intending to take action regarding his alcohol use in the immediate future. Which stage of change is he in?
   a. Contemplation
   b. Action
   c. Preparation
   d. Precontemplation

10. EBP is defined as
   a. a system bringing to bear the best available scientific evidence to clinical decision-making.
   b. a process for translating decision-making into individualized patient care.
   c. the assessment of risks and benefits of treatment versus nontreatment.
   d. the use of critical thinking to determine priorities in diagnosis and treatment.

5 The Health Record

LEARNING OBJECTIVES

After studying Chapter 5 in the textbook and completing this section of the laboratory manual, students should be able to:
1. Discuss the characteristics and multiple functions of the Electronic Health Record (EHR).
2. Describe reasons for maintaining clear and accurate records.
3. Discuss various components of the problem-oriented medical record set out in the terminology review below.
4. Organize data in appropriate system sections of the history.
5. Delineate methods for documenting the location and description of findings.

TERMINOLOGY REVIEW

Check your understanding of terminology related to recording information. Using the space provided, write the word or phrase from the list next to the appropriate descriptor.

Chief concern
Comprehensive health history and physical
   examination
Episodic illness visit
Family history
History of present illness
Information integrity
OLDCARTS mnemonic

Past medical history
Personal and social history
Plan
Problem list
Problem-oriented medical record (POMR)
Subjective, Objective, Assessment, Plan (SOAP)

1. _____: a format for recording health history and physical examination findings by documenting the problem assessment process.

2. _____: scenario in which a patient seeks care for an acute problem, which is usually rapidly resolved.

3. _____: onset, location, duration, character, aggravating factors, relieving factors, temporal factors, and severity of symptoms.

4. _____: dependability of information, that is, accuracy, consistency, and reliability of information content.

5. _____: a brief description of the patient's main reason for seeking care, stated verbatim in quotation marks.

6. _____: part of the medical record that includes cultural background, birthplace, education, family, marital status, general life satisfaction, hobbies, sources of stress, and religious practices.

7. _____: a list of interventions divided into three categories—diagnosis, treatment, and patient education—based on each problem in the problem list.

8. _____: record that must include all data collected, both positive and negative, that contribute to the examiner's assessment.

9. _____: information about general health over the patient's lifetime as well as disabilities and functional limitations as the patient perceives them.

10. _____: a detailed description of all symptoms that may be related to the chief concern; describes the concern for problem chronologically, dating events, and symptoms.

11. _____: a pedigree with at least three generations and information about major health or genetic disorders.

12. _____: a running log of problem number, date of onset, description of problem, and date the problem was resolved.

APPLICATION TO CLINICAL PRACTICE

Concepts Application 1

Fill in the blanks in the following statements, selecting appropriate terms from the list below.

Subjective	Chief concern
SOAP	Objective
Illustration	Health history
POMR	Incremental grading
	Physical examination

1. _____ data are collected during the history and are based on patient reports.

2. A brief description of the patient's main reason for seeking healthcare is referred to as the _____.

3. _____ is a format used to document health history notes, especially for care beyond the initial evaluation.

4. The use of stick people to document findings is an example of using a(n) _____.

5. _____ data are collected while conducting the physical examination.

6. _____ is the use of recorded numbers to represent findings by variable degrees.

7. _____ is a widely accepted medical record format consisting of six components.

8. _____ is the part of the record where information from a patient interview is recorded.

9. Clinical findings are recorded during the _____.

Concepts Application 2

Develop a patient problem list based on the following information.

A patient comes to the clinic because of back pain. She indicates that this pain started in January 2021 while she was moving some rocks in her garden. Other pertinent aspects of her history include insulin-dependent diabetes mellitus since 2005, which she says she has never really had under control, and cholecystitis, for which she had a cholecystectomy in May 2001. She has a family history of atherosclerotic heart disease and chronic renal failure.

Problem #	Onset	Problem	Date Resolved
1.	January 2021	Low back pain	Ongoing
2.			
3.			
4.			
5.			

A 37-year-old woman has been interviewed for a health history. Her family history is contained in the following paragraph. Below the paragraph, draw a pedigree for her family history using the information provided.

The patient is married. Her husband is 43 years old. They have a 12-year-old son, an 11-year-old daughter, and a 10-year-old son, all in good health. The patient has a 42-year-old brother and three sisters, 40, 36, and 32 years of age. All of her siblings are in good health. Both of her parents are alive. Her 70-year-old father has mild emphysema and is an only child. Her mother is 66 years old and has hypertension. Her mother has three siblings: the oldest is a brother who is 74 years old and has glaucoma, another brother is 72 years old and is in good health, and a sister who is 69 years old and has osteoarthritis. All of the patient's grandparents are deceased. Her paternal grandfather died at the age of 89 years of prostate cancer. Her paternal grandmother died of congestive heart failure at the age of 91 years. Her maternal grandfather died at the age of 86 years of prostate cancer, and her maternal grandmother died at 96 years of "old age."

CLINICAL REASONING

1. The onset of a "new" symptom should be thoroughly documented. Describe what the mnemonic device "OLD-CARTS" refers to regarding documentation of a symptom.

   O:

   L:

   D:

   C:

   A:

   R:

   T:

   S:

2. While examining a patient, you note a mass. What characteristics should be described when documenting any organ, mass, or lesion?

Patient Safety Consideration

The Joint Commission has identified "improving communications among caregivers" as a patient safety goal. What are two major ways in which you can support this goal when you are recording patient information?

CONTENT REVIEW QUESTIONS

Multiple Choice

Circle the best answer for each of the following questions.

1. Which of the following examples illustrates a vague or nondescriptive term?
   a. "Skin color is normal."
   b. "Skin turgor is elastic."
   c. "Skin is thin and smooth."
   d. "Skin is warm and dry."

2. How are "normal findings" best documented?
   a. Write "normal" or "within normal limits" on the documentation form.
   b. Write "NA" (not applicable) on the documentation sheet.
   c. Because documentation focuses on abnormal findings, do not write anything for normal findings.
   d. Document what was actually assessed in specific terms.

3. One way that a health history for an infant differs from that of an adult is the inclusion of
   a. nutritional history.
   b. chief concern.
   c. prenatal information.
   d. personal social information.

4. If a mistake is made in a paper patient record, it is suggested that a line be drawn through the mistake so that it is still legible and then signed. The basis for this action is related to the fact that
   a. no errors are allowed.
   b. the chart is a legal document.
   c. a pen is messy when used to obliterate writing.
   d. others may want to read what your first impressions were.

5. Which of the following statements is true regarding use of abbreviations?
   a. Use of any abbreviations is fine as long as you can interpret them.
   b. Abbreviations should be used as much as possible to reduce time and space needed for documentation.
   c. Abbreviations should be avoided because they are not considered acceptable.
   d. Use only universally accepted abbreviations for documentation.

6. The examiner can substantially reduce the possibility of legal problems by
   a. maintaining clear medical records.
   b. using the SOAP format to document all entries.
   c. using a POMR.
   d. drawing genograms in the patient record.

7. Which of the following information belongs in a family history?
   a. Chronic illness
   b. Current problems
   c. Genetic disorders
   d. Personal data

8. You are taking a health history of your patient, who presented with a lump in her left breast. When you are asking about problems, your patient reports constipation over the past 5 or 6 months. This would be documented in
   a. chief complaint.
   b. past medical history.
   c. review of systems.
   d. assessment.

9. Your patient presents to the office with a chief concern of shoulder pain that he reports as stabbing. In using the mnemonic OLDCARTS, this is noted as
   a. character.
   b. duration.
   c. location.
   d. onset.

10. Which statement complies with recommended guidelines for documentation in a patient's record?
    a. Skin turgor is good.
    b. Patient appears anxious.
    c. Patient says she "feels down."
    d. Vital signs are within normal range.

6 Vital Signs and Pain Assessment

After studying Chapter 6 in the textbook and completing this section of the laboratory manual, students should be able to:

1. Explain the assessment of vital signs and pain in adult patients as well as in special populations, such as infants, children, and older adults.
2. Describe the techniques to assess vital signs, including temperature, pulse, respirations, and blood pressure.
3. Discuss the use of pain assessment scales in the history and physical examination of pain.
4. Evaluate vital sign findings that deviate from normal.
5. Analyze the impact of pain on physiologic responses.
6. Describe a focused history and physical examination in a patient experiencing an alteration in vital signs or pain.

TERMINOLOGY REVIEW

Check your understanding of terminology related to assessment of vital signs. Using the space provided, write the word or phrase from the list next to the appropriate descriptor.

Blood pressure (BP)	**Pulse rate**
Complex regional pain syndrome	**Pulse pressure**
FLACC Behavioral Pain Assessment Scale	**Pyrexia**
Korotkoff sounds	**Respiratory rate**
Neonatal infant pain scale	**Shivering**
Neuropathic pain	**Tachypnea**
PAINAD	**Temperature**
	Wong/Baker faces rating scale

1. _____: faster than normal respiratory rate.

2. _____: the fever response triggered by prostaglandins.

3. _____: the force of the blood against the wall of an artery as the ventricles of the heart contract and relax.

4. _____: tool for scoring pain behaviors in non-communicative older adults with dementia.

5. _____: used to assess procedural pain in infants up to 6 weeks of age.

6. _____: a form of chronic pain caused by a primary lesion or by dysfunction of the central nervous system that persists longer than expected after healing.

7. _____: this assessment is most commonly performed by oral, rectal, axillary, tympanic, or forehead routes.

8. _____: the presence of regional pain beyond the original nerve injury with motor, sensory, and autonomic changes after a predominately traumatic, noxious event, with or without specific nerve injury.

9. _____: a pain scale for non-verbal children.

10. _____: palpated over an artery close to the body surface that lies over bones.

11. _____: turbulence of blood flow in the artery.

12. _____: assessed by inspecting the rise and fall of the chest; the expected adult rate is 12 to 20 breaths/min.

13. _____: a pain scale for children using a scale of 0 to 5.

14. _____: rapid contraction and relaxation of the skeletal muscles.

15. _____: the difference between the systolic and diastolic pressures.

APPLICATION TO CLINICAL PRACTICE

Clinical Case Study 1

A 41-year-old woman presents to the clinic with a fever. She does not have any past medical illnesses. She does not smoke or drink alcohol.

1. What characteristics of her fever would you ask about?

2. What associated symptoms would you ask about?

3. What medication would you ask about?

Clinical Case Study 2

A 65-year-old woman is hospitalized for acute back pain. Her history includes carpal tunnel syndrome, colitis, and osteoarthritis.

1. What pain findings would you expect for each problem listed below? (Write your answers in the space provided in the right-hand column.)

Diagnosis	Pain Findings
Acute pain	
Carpal tunnel syndrome	
Colitis	
Osteoarthritis	

CLINICAL REASONING

Clinical Reasoning Case Study 1

A 65-year-old man who is brought to the office for hypertension follow-up. On presentation, his BP is 148/92 mm Hg and pulse is 56 beats/min.

1. What is the most common cause of hypertension in elderly adults?

2. What age-related factor may be responsible for a pulse rate of 56 beats/minute?

Clinical Reasoning Case Study 2

An 85-year-old patient presents to your clinic with a complaint of "awful soreness" in the abdomen.

1. What physical signs would you expect to find during a physical examination?

2. When asked for further description, the patient identifies the soreness as cramping sensations. What would you anticipate the underlying condition to be?

Patient Safety Consideration

A patient receives intravenous morphine for pain at 11:10 AM. You know that the peak effect of the drug should occur in 10 to 20 minutes, so you plan to assess the patient at 11:20 and again at 11:30. How does this plan contribute to the patient safety?

CONTENT REVIEW QUESTIONS

Multiple Choice
Circle the best answer for each of the following questions:

1. Which is an important consideration when assessing pain in a 32-year-old postoperative patient?
   a. Previous experiences with pain will influence both pain perception and interpretation.
   b. Intensity is the characteristic of pain that is most easily determined.
   c. Dementia can occur as a response to excessive pain.
   d. Pain is an objective symptom; thus, validation is not necessary.

2. When obtaining a patient's blood pressure, how can the examiner protect against an incorrect reading because of the auscultatory gap?
   a. Position the patient with the limb used for the blood pressure measurement at heart level.
   b. Deflate the cuff at a rate of 2 to 3 mm Hg per second.
   c. Use the popliteal rather than the radial artery.
   d. Palpate the systolic pressure prior to taking the blood pressure with a stethoscope.

3. Which term is commonly used by a child expressing pain?
   a. Cutting
   b. Hurt
   c. Sting
   d. Stabbing

4. A 32-year-old patient is admitted in severe pain with a fractured right ankle after an automobile accident. Which assessment finding would be **unexpected** given the painful nature of the injury?
   a. Facial distortions, such as grimacing
   b. Changes in vital signs, including BP and pulse
   c. Increase in attention span and talking
   d. Splinting of her leg and ankle

5. At about what age is a child able to respond to a pediatric pain scale?
   a. 3 years old
   b. 7 years old
   c. 11 years old
   d. 14 years old

6. The CRIES scale would appropriately be used when assessing which of the following patients?
   a. A premature newborn in respiratory distress
   b. A 2-month-old postoperative infant
   c. A year-old baby with Down syndrome
   d. A toddler with a seizure disorder

7. When you are completing an assessment on a patient with pain, it is important to
   a. do a complete assessment to check for referred pain.
   b. learn the patient's customary terminology.
   c. medicate the patient before the assessment so as not to hurt the patient.
   d. always use a nonverbal patient pain scale.

8. The gold standard in pain assessment is the patient's
   a. nonverbal communication.
   b. perception of his or her own pain.
   c. vital signs.
   d. fear of addiction.

9. A 51-year-old patient is admitted with burning, shock-like pain in the left hand. This finding suggests a problem involving which type of tissue?
   a. Nerve
   b. Cardiac
   c. Bone
   d. Soft tissue

10. On what basis does an examiner determine the correct size of a BP cuff for an adult?
    a. Ratio of cuff length to limb length
    b. Number of times the cuff will wrap around the limb
    c. Percent of limb covered by the cuff
    d. Relationship between cuff bladder size and limb size

11. How is a BP reading affected if an adult cuff is used on a small child?
    a. BP reading will be falsely low.
    b. BP reading will be artificially high.
    c. Systolic reading will be falsely high and the diastolic falsely low.
    d. BP readings are not affected provided the cuff is properly positioned.

12. Assessment using the PAINAD tool should be done when
    a. some patient activity, such as turning or transferring, is in progress.
    b. the patient first awakens in the morning.
    c. the environment is quiet and free of distractions.
    d. the patient is cooperative and not agitated.

13. The expected respiratory rate for children age 6 years old is between
    a. 20 to 40 breaths/min.
    b. 20 to 30 breaths/min.
    c. 16 to 22 breaths/min.
    d. 12 to 20 breaths/min.

14. You are assessing a 10-year-old boy. Which pulse rate is within the normal range for a child of this age?
    a. 68 beats/min
    b. 74 beats/min
    c. 82 beats/min
    d. 96 beats/min

15. A 14 year-old boy weighing 108 pounds is having a routine physical examination. His BP is 138/78 mm Hg. Which factor must you consider as a potential cause of his elevated systolic BP?
    a. Anxiety
    b. Gender
    c. Age
    d. Weight

16. Potential causes of secondary hypertension include all of the following **except**
    a. increased water intake.
    b. renal artery stenosis.
    c. thyroid disorders.
    d. coarctation of the aorta.

17. When checking a patient's respiratory rate, which guideline should the examiner follow?
    a. Ask the patient to breathe quietly through the mouth.
    b. Keep the patient unaware that respirations are being counted.
    c. Place a hand on the patient's back, midway between the shoulder blades.
    d. Count the number of times the patient inhales in 30 seconds and multiply by two.

18. Which is the best method for checking the patient's pulse?
    a. Count for 30 seconds and multiply by 2.
    b. Count the pulse for 20 seconds and multiply by 3.
    c. Count the pulse for 15 seconds and multiply by 4.
    d. Count the pulse for 10 seconds and multiply by 6.

19. Which is the effect of a too-loose cuff on blood pressure measurement?
    a. Absence of Korotkoff sounds
    b. Inaccurate diastolic reading
    c. Falsely elevated systolic reading
    d. Prolonged auscultatory gap

20. Which blood pressure change occurring when a patient goes from a sitting to a standing position is indicative of orthostatic hypotension?
    a. Systolic BP drop greater than 5 mm Hg and a diastolic drop of 5 mm Hg.
    b. Systolic BP drop greater than 10 mm Hg and a diastolic drop of 10 mm Hg.
    c. Systolic BP drop greater than 20 mm Hg and a diastolic drop of 10 mm Hg.
    d. Systolic BP drop greater than 20 mm Hg and a diastolic drop of 20 mm Hg.

7 Mental Status

LEARNING OBJECTIVES

After studying Chapter 7 in the textbook and completing this section of the laboratory manual, students should be able to:
1. Identify aspects of an interview that facilitate mental status examination.
2. Describe techniques to assess mental status in the following areas: physical appearance, cognitive abilities, emotional stability, speech, and language skills.
3. Recognize mental status findings that deviate from expected findings.
4. Compare and contrast common conditions affecting mental status.
5. Identify conditions affecting mental status in various age groups.

TERMINOLOGY REVIEW

Check your understanding of terminology related to mental status. Using the space provided, write the word or phrase from the list next to the appropriate descriptor.

Affect	**Dysarthria**
Aphasia	**Dysphonia**
Apraxia	**Glasgow Coma Scale**
Broca	**Hallucination**
Cognitive	**Insults**
Coherence	**Judgment**
Comprehension	**Wernicke**

1. _____: events in the brain—such as trauma, infection, or chemical imbalance—that can damage brain cells that may result in serious permanent dysfunction in mental status.

2. _____: clear, logical flow of ideas, intentions, and perceptions.

3. _____: area of the temporal lobe that permits comprehension of spoken and written language.

4. _____: the inability to translate an intention into action that is unrelated to paralysis or lack of comprehension; may indicate a cerebral disorder.

5. _____: a disorder of voice volume, quality, or pitch.

6. _____: an emotional response or feeling.

7. _____: a scale used to assess the function of the cerebral cortex and brainstem and to quantify consciousness.

8. _____: area associated with speech formation.

9. _____: a speech disorder that can be receptive (understanding language) or expressive (speaking language); it may be indicated by hesitations and other speech rhythm disturbances, omission of syllables or words, word transposition, circumlocutions, and neologisms.

10. _____: the ability to reason.

11. _____: pertaining to mental processes of memory, judgment, and reasoning; cognitive impairment is characterized by a loss of memory, confusion, and inappropriate affect.

12. _____: a motor speech disorder defect associated with many conditions of the nervous system such as stroke, inebriation, cerebral palsy, and Parkinson disease.

13. _____: capacity of the mind to understand; demonstrated by an ability to follow simple instructions.

14. _____: a sensory experience not due to external stimulus.

APPLICATION TO CLINICAL PRACTICE

Matching
Match each mental status term with its corresponding definition.

Definition	Mental Status Term
_____ 1. Feelings of helplessness	a. Mood lability
_____ 2. Apprehension	b. Anxiety
_____ 3. Excessive happiness	c. Flat affect
_____ 4. Rapid shift of emotions	d. Depression
_____ 5. Lack of emotional response	e. Irritability
_____ 6. Annoyed response to stimulus	f. Euphoria

Clinical Concepts Application
List ways that the following aspects of cognitive abilities might be assessed during examination. For each assessment, briefly describe how a patient's response would be evaluated.

1. Attention

2. Recent Memory

3. Judgment

4. Abstract reasoning

5. Thought processes and content

A 78-year-old woman is brought to the geriatric clinic by her son and daughter-in-law. Her son tells the examiner that his father passed away 5 months ago and, ever since then, his mother has "gone downhill." He indicates that his mother is no longer keeping her house clean or cooking appropriate meals. Also, her personal hygiene habits have changed dramatically. She has lost interest in getting her hair done and she no longer likes to get dressed for the day.

He tells the examiner, "When I suggest a retirement home, she becomes very angry and tells me to mind my own business. I am just worried about Mom, and I want to make sure she is well cared for." During this conversation, the patient sits quietly. She interjects only to say, "I have taken care of you, your brother, and your father. Now, all of a sudden, you think I am helpless and want to lock me away." She appears clean, although her hair is matted, and her clothes are badly wrinkled and do not match. Her speech is clear, but her overall affect is very dull. She does not make eye contact with her son or the examiner. A physical examination demonstrates normal bodily functioning consistent with her age group.

1. Which data deviate from normal findings, suggesting altered mental health?

2. What additional questions could the examiner ask to clarify the patient's symptoms?

3. What additional physical examination, if any, should the examiner complete?

4. The patient's symptoms are consistent with what condition affecting mental health?

CLINICAL REASONING

1. How are depression, delirium, and dementia differentiated?

2. What is the expected effect of aging on cognitive function in a healthy adult?

Patient Safety Consideration

As part of your assessment, you ask a patient who appears depressed if he has actually had any thoughts of killing himself. The patient responds that, 5 days ago, he had started to rig his car so he could die of carbon monoxide poisoning but then he "turned chicken." What actions do you take?

Multiple Choice

Circle the best answer for each of the following questions:

1. A patient's inability to follow simple instructions could indicate which of the following findings?
   a. Dysphonia
   b. Amnesia
   c. Aphasia
   d. Depression

2. A patient scores a 3 on the Mini-Cog Assessment Instrument for Dementia. What does this score indicate?
   a. Advanced dementia
   b. Early dementia
   c. Need for further evaluation
   d. Negative screen for dementia

3. The examiner asks the patient to complete this statement: "A bird is to air as a fish is to...." This is an example of what type of testing?
   a. Calculation
   b. Analogy
   c. Judgment
   d. Mood and feelings

4. Assume that the patient's response to the examiner in question 3 is "scales." What does this response likely reflect?
   a. Left cerebral hemisphere lesion
   b. Depression
   c. Eating disorder
   d. Aphasia

5. Which type of assessment should be used to evaluate the mental status of a patient with head trauma?
   a. PHQ
   b. Perceptual distortion assessment
   c. Glasgow Coma Scale
   d. Functional assessment

6. Which of the following indicates possible cognitive impairment?
   a. Ability to complete personal care without assistance
   b. Suspiciousness or inappropriate affect
   c. Articulate communication
   d. Prudent behavior and calm demeanor

7. A 65-year-old woman is brought to the clinic by family members, who report that they have noticed a change in her mental abilities over the past 2 weeks. Normally, they say, she is independent, intelligent, and very socially oriented. Her medical history is unremarkable except for congestive heart failure, for which she takes digoxin. She has had no major changes in her health. What question would be the most important for the examiner to ask this woman's family?
   a. "Is there a family history of Alzheimer disease?"
   b. "How much alcohol does she drink in an average week?"
   c. "When was her digoxin blood level last checked?"
   d. "Did you know that mental function begins to decline after the age of 60?"

8. A patient who has difficulty writing or drawing is most likely to have which condition?
   a. Temporal lobe damage
   b. Peripheral neuropathy
   c. Organic brain syndrome
   d. Psychiatric hallucinations

9. A mother brings her 18-month-old son to the clinic. She states that the child rarely talks or smiles or makes eye contact. She has also noticed that he does not like to be held. She says his motor development seems to be normal. These symptoms are consistent with what condition?
   a. Dementia
   b. Autistic disorder
   c. ADHD
   d. Delirium

10. A patient with Alzheimer disease classically displays which of the following?
    a. Alternating periods of mania and stupor
    b. Hallucinations and decorticate posturing
    c. Disintegration of personality
    d. Rapid onset of symptoms

8 Growth and Nutrition

LEARNING OBJECTIVES

After studying Chapter 8 in the textbook and completing this section of the laboratory manual, students should be able to:
1. Recognize anatomic and physiologic factors that influence growth and nutrition.
2. Identify interview methods to gather data pertinent to growth, development, and nutrition.
3. Describe tools and instruments used to assess developmental achievement and nutrition.
4. Identify expected findings relevant to growth, development, and nutrition throughout the life span.
5. Describe variations in findings that may be considered within normal range.

TERMINOLOGY REVIEW

Check your understanding of terminology related to growth and nutrition. Using the space provided, write the word or phrase from the list next to the appropriate descriptor.

Ballard gestational age assessment	**Obesity**
Body mass index	**Pica**
Failure to thrive	**Recumbent length**
Gestational age	**Sexual maturity rating**
Head circumference	**Twenty-four-hour recall**
Macronutrients	**Velocity**
Micronutrients	**Waist-to-height ratio**

1. _____: a parameter of growth calculated by charting changes in height over a time interval.

2. _____: nutrients required by the body in large amounts (carbohydrates, fats, and proteins).

3. _____: nonnutritive eating.

4. _____: a marker used to determine a child's pubertal development.

5. _____: an assessment tool that evaluates six physical and six neuromuscular characteristics within 36 hours of birth to establish or confirm the newborn's gestational age.

6. _____: a measurement that should be obtained on each visit until a child reaches 2–3 years of age.

7. _____: a measure of fat distribution by body type.

8. _____: the most common method used to assess nutritional status and total body fat.

9. _____: vitamins, minerals, and electrolytes required and stored by the body in small amounts.

10. _____: an indicator of a newborn's maturity.

11. _____: length of an infant from birth to 24 months of age measured in the supine position on the measuring device.

12. _____: falling one or more standard deviations off growth curve pattern; below the fifth percentile for weight and height.

13. _____: excessive proportion of total body fat.

14. _____: method for obtaining a food intake history in which the patient is asked to list all foods, beverages, and snacks ingested during the past 24 hours.

APPLICATION TO CLINICAL PRACTICE

Clinical Case Study 1

A 43-year-old man presents with a loss of energy, loss of appetite, and loss of weight. He states that he used to maintain a steady weight of 172 pounds but that over the past 9 months he has gradually lost weight. He is 5 feet, 9 inches tall and currently weighs 142 pounds.

1. Calculate the patient's current body mass index (BMI). (Refer to Box 8.4 in the textbook for help).

   Current BMI: _____

2. What was his previous BMI (before his weight loss)?

   Previous BMI: _____

Personal Food Record

1. Explore the various 24-hour recall tools available online. Select one and complete it for yourself.

Personal Food Assessment

Visit the ChooseMyPlate.gov website to create a Daily Food Plan based on your age, gender, weight, height, and physical activity.

Personal Analysis of Nutritional Needs

1. Analyze the data you have gathered during your personal food record and personal food assessment above. Compare your results with the suggested daily servings from the ChooseMyPlate.gov website.

A One-Day (24-Hour) Record of Food Intake

NAME _____   DATE OF RECORD _____

BREAKFAST   Time Eaten _____

Food/Beverage	Type and/or Method of Preparation (List Ingredients)	Amount
MILK		
FRUIT fresh, canned, sweetened, etc.		
CEREAL _____ with milk _____ with sugar _____ other	Brand _____	
BREAD _____ margarine/butter _____ mayonnaise _____ other	White _____ Brown _____	
EGGS		
MEAT or OTHER PROTEIN		
BEVERAGE _____ with milk _____ with sugar _____ other		
OTHER FOODS		

Did you eat a mid-morning snack?   Yes _____   No _____   If yes, time? _____
(List foods and beverages eaten.)

_____

_____

NOON MEAL   Time Eaten _____

Food/Beverage	Type and/or Method of Preparation (List Ingredients)	Amount
SOUP		
BREAD _____ margarine/butter _____ mayonnaise _____ other	White _____ Brown _____	
_____ MEAT _____ EGG _____ FISH _____ CHEESE		

VEGETABLES
_____ cooked
_____ raw
_____ topping/seasoning
    (butter, white
    sauce, cheese
    sauce, etc.)		

SALAD _____ dressing (brand, etc.)		
FRUIT fresh, canned, sweetened, etc.		
MILK		
BEVERAGE _____ with milk _____ with sugar _____ other		
DESSERT		
OTHER FOODS		

Did you eat an afternoon snack?   Yes _____   No _____   If yes, time? _____
(List foods and beverages eaten.)

_____

_____

EVENING MEAL   Time Eaten _____

Food/Beverage	Type and/or Method of Preparation (List Ingredients)	Amount
MAIN DISH _____ meat _____ cheese _____ poultry _____ other protein _____ pasta _____ rice		

VEGETABLES
_____ cooked
_____ raw
_____ topping/seasoning
    (butter, white
    sauce, cheese
    sauce, etc.)		

SALAD _____ dressing (brand, etc.)		
BREAD _____ margarine/butter _____ mayonnaise _____ other	White _____ Brown _____	
FRUIT fresh, canned, sweetened, etc.		
MILK		
BEVERAGE _____ with milk _____ with sugar _____ other		
DESSERT		
OTHER FOODS		

Did you eat an evening snack? Yes _____   No _____   If yes, time? _____
(List foods and beverages eaten.)

_____

_____

Modified from Burke B: The dietary history as a tool in research, *J Am Dietic Assoc* 23:1044–1046, 1947.

1. Normal growth and development require the interaction of many hormones. For each of the following hormones, describe its activity in the body.
   a. Growth hormone

   b. Growth hormone–releasing hormone (GHRH)

   c. Somatostatin

   d. Insulin-like growth factor 1 (IGF-1)

2. Growth at puberty is dependent on the interaction of hormones. For each of the following hormones, describe its activity in the body.
   a. Sex steroids (androgens)

   b. Testosterone

   c. Estrogen

3. What is the role of leptin in growth of the body?

Matching

Match each description with the hormone disorder that it represents.

Characteristic	Hormone Disorder
_____ 1. A 16-year-old female with absence of sexual development; also has short stature and increased carrying angle of the elbows.	a. Acromegaly
_____ 2. Woman with a round face, reddish purple striae, and fat accumulation in the lower posterior cervical area.	b. Adolescence
	c. Cushing syndrome
_____ 3. A 5-year-old girl with pubertal changes.	d. Hydrocephalus
_____ 4. Child with pronounced head enlargement and increased intracranial pressure.	e. Precocious puberty
_____ 5. Half of an individual's ideal weight gained during this period.	f. Turner syndrome
_____ 6. A 60-year-old man with exaggerated facial features and massive hands.	

Patient Safety Consideration

Interactions between foods and medications can threaten patient safety. Mixing certain foods with certain medications can interfere with the effectiveness of the medications or can exacerbate the side effects. Research food–drug interactions and list examples to be alert for when completing a history and physical examination on a patient.

CONTENT REVIEW QUESTIONS

Multiple Choice

Circle the best answer for each of the following questions.

1. A 38-year-old woman is 5 feet 7 inches tall and weighs 163 pounds. Based on these measurements, the examiner assesses total body fat using the
   a. upper-to-lower body segment ratio.
   b. arm span.
   c. waist-to-hip circumference ratio.
   d. body mass index.

2. The body mass index of a patient who is 5 feet 3 inches tall and weighs 142 pounds would be
   a. 21.
   b. 25.2.
   c. 27.
   d. 29.5.

3. With a BMI of 22.6, you would consider a patient to be
   a. underweight.
   b. of normal weight.
   c. overweight.
   d. obese.

4. The majority of brain growth is completed by
   a. 1 year of age.
   b. 2 years of age.
   c. 3 years of age.
   d. 7 years of age.

5. A child has an arm span that measures greater than his height. This finding is consistent with what condition?
   a. Turner syndrome
   b. Marfan syndrome
   c. Acromegaly
   d. Failure to thrive

6. Which assessment data do you need to calculate a Sexual Maturity Rating (SMR) for a 13-year-old female patient?
   a. Height, weight, and age of menarche
   b. Ages at which breast stage 4 and pubic hair stage 5 were reached
   c. Age of peak height velocity and average stage of breast and pubic hair development
   d. Stage of breast development and stage of pubic hair development

7. To accurately assess height velocity, the examiner must measure a child's height at
   a. 6-month intervals.
   b. 12-month intervals.
   c. 18-month intervals.
   d. 24-month intervals.

8. A pregnant patient has a prepregnancy body mass index of 22.4. The examiner expects this patient's weight gain during pregnancy to fall into which weight range?
   a. Less than 20 pounds
   b. 20 to 26 pounds
   c. 25 to 35 pounds
   d. 40 to 50 pounds

9. You ask an 82-year-old patient to keep a food diary to aid in assessing the adequacy of her diet. Which is an appropriate instruction to provide?
   a. Keep the diary for 3 days. Start tomorrow morning at breakfast and end before breakfast on Friday.
   b. Make a list of what and how much you eat or drink at each meal for the next week.
   c. Keep a record of everything you eat and drink over the weekend. Be sure to include snacks and alcohol.
   d. Write down what and how much of everything you eat and drink for four days, at least one of which is a weekend day.

10. To assess and monitor growth, the examiner makes routine measurements of an infant's weight, length, and which of the following?
    a. Head circumference
    b. Hip-to-toe length
    c. Forearm length
    d. Chest circumference

11. A 4-month-old infant is brought to the clinic. At birth, the baby weighed 6 pounds, 8 ounces. If the baby is gaining weight at the desired rate, the examiner should expect the baby to now weigh
    a. 9 pounds.
    b. 11 pounds.
    c. 13 pounds.
    d. 15 pounds.

12. Which hormone has a key role in regulating body fat mass and is thought to be a trigger for puberty?
    a. Leptin
    b. Androgen
    c. Estrogen
    d. Growth hormone

13. A dietary assessment is performed by
    a. comparing established eating habits with the recommended dietary allowances.
    b. asking the patient to fill out a food pyramid.
    c. comparing the recommended dietary allowances to the U.S. Department of Agriculture MyPlate.
    d. asking the patient to do a 24-hour dietary recall.

14. Which position would you ask a 14-year-old male patient to assume in order for you to assess his pubertal development?
    a. Sitting
    b. Standing
    c. Lying supine
    d. Knee–chest

15. A 22-year-old patient presents for a routine physical examination. As part of her history, she states that she has been on a vegan diet for 14 months. Based on this information, you would be most concerned about a possible deficiency in which two nutrients?
    a. Calcium and vitamin B_{12}
    b. Protein and iron
    c. Vitamin D and phosphorus
    d. Fat and vitamin A

9 Skin, Hair, and Nails

LEARNING OBJECTIVES

After studying Chapter 9 in the textbook and completing this section of the laboratory manual, students should be able to:

1. Conduct a history related of skin, hair, and nails.
2. Discuss examination techniques for skin, hair, and nails.
3. Identify normal age and condition variations of the skin, hair, and nails.
4. Recognize findings that deviate from expected results.
5. Relate symptoms or clinical findings to common pathologic conditions.

TERMINOLOGY REVIEW

Check your understanding of terminology related to skin assessment. Using the space provided, write the word or phrase from the list next to the appropriate descriptor.

Acrocyanosis	**Nevus**
Alopecia	**Petechiae**
Annular	**Plaque**
Chloasma	**Reticulate**
Confluent	**Salmon patches (stork bites)**
Dermatomal	**Sebum**
Ecchymosis	**Serpiginous**
Generalized	**Stellate**
Keloid	**Telangiectasias**
Lanugo	**Vernix caseosa**
Melanin	**Vesicle**
Morbilliform	

1. _____: round, active margins with central clearing.

2. _____: referring to lesions that run together.

3. _____: widely distributed or present in several areas simultaneously.

4. _____: a mole that varies in size and degree of pigmentation.

5. _____: a fluid-filled and elevated, but superficial, skin lesion.

6. _____: a bluish discoloration of the hands and feet that may be present at birth and may persist for several days or longer if the newborn is kept in cool ambient temperatures.

7. _____: fine, silky hair of newborns found on the shoulders and back.

8. _____: tiny, flat, purple, or red spots on the skin surface resulting from minute hemorrhages within the dermal layer smaller than 0.5 cm in diameter.

9. _____: refers to maculopapular lesions that become confluent on the face and body.

10. _____: hair loss.

11. _____: permanently dilated, small blood vessels consisting of venules or arterioles.

12. _____: hyperpigmentation that occurs in pregnant women and is found on the forehead, cheeks, bridge of the nose, and chin; it is blotchy and symmetric.

13. _____: flat, deep-pink, localized areas usually seen on the midforehead, eyelids, upper lip, and back of the neck in a newborn.

14. _____: a discoloration produced by injury.

15. _____: a lipid substance that keeps skin and hair from drying out.

16. _____: a type of skin lesion common in patients with psoriasis.

17. _____: referring to a lesion that follows a nerve or segment of the body.

18. _____: irregularly shaped, elevated, progressively enlarging, and hypertrophied scar.

19. _____: referring to a star-shaped lesion.

20. _____: synthesized in the stratum germinativum by melanocytes and is the pigment that gives skin its color.

21. _____: a mixture of sebum and cornified epidermis that covers the infant's body at birth.

22. _____: referring to a lesion with a netlike or lacy appearance.

23. _____: referring to lesions that appear to occur in a wavy line.

APPLICATION TO CLINICAL PRACTICE

Anatomy Review

Identify structures on the diagram of the nail by writing the correct term in the blank next to the corresponding letter.

a. _____

b. _____

c. _____

d. _____

e. _____

Identify the type of secondary lesion shown in each illustration below. For each type of lesion, give one or more common examples.

	Type of Lesion	Examples
1.		
2.		
3.		
4.		

Matching 1

Match each type of lesion with its corresponding description or the condition with which the lesion is commonly associated.

Description or Associated Condition	Type of Lesion
_____ 1. Chickenpox	a. Papule
_____ 2. Insect bite	b. Macule
_____ 3. Impetigo	c. Vesicle
_____ 4. Chronic atopic dermatitis	d. Tumor
_____ 5. Lipoma	e. Pustule
_____ 6. Blister	f. Patch
_____ 7. Wart	g. Lichenification
_____ 8. Port-wine stain	h. Wheal
_____ 9. Petechiae	i. Bulla

Matching 2

Match the dermatologic finding with its appropriate description:

Dermatologic Finding	Description
_____ 1. Palmar erythema	a. Contagious staphylococcal or streptococcal infection of the epidermis
_____ 2. Sebaceous hyperplasia	b. Yellowish, flattened papules with central depression
_____ 3. Solar lentigenes	c. Irregular, gray-brown macules that occur in sun-exposed areas that can range in size from a few millimeters to over a centimeter.
_____ 4. Impetigo	d. Diffuse redness over palmar surface during pregnancy

Matching 3

Match each part of the skin anatomy with the area in which it is found. (Note: Letters will be used more than once.)

Skin Anatomy	Area Found
_____ 1. Stratum corneum	a. Epidermis
_____ 2. Autonomic motor nerves	b. Dermis
_____ 3. Cellular stratum	c. Hypodermis
_____ 4. Keratin cells	
_____ 5. Reticulum fibers	
_____ 6. Subcutaneous layer	
_____ 7. Stratum germinativum	
_____ 8. Layer that generates heat	

A 74-year-old man comes to the clinic for a "routine checkup." Listed below are data collected by the examiner on the patient's skin, hair, and nails.

INTERVIEW DATA

The patient denies any specific complaints except that he has some nonpainful sores on his legs that "don't seem to want to heal."

EXAMINATION DATA

Hair distribution: Full head of hair that is coarse and thinning. No areas of balding noted. Hair color is gray.

Overall appearance of skin: Skin is pale pink, thin, and dry, with flaking and tenting present.

Face and neck: Pigmented, raised, warty lesions (seborrheic keratosis) noted on face. Three cutaneous tags noted on neck. Several senile lentigines lesions noted on neck and face.

Chest and abdomen: 1-mm, tiny, bright-red, round papules (cherry angiomas) noted on chest. Angular surgical scar noted in right upper abdomen.

Extremities: Legs and ankles have areas of erythematous, scaling, and weeping patches. Legs slightly edematous. No hair growth noted on legs. Upper arms: Skin very thin and dry; several senile lentigines noted on arms bilaterally.

Nails: Nails are yellowish and thick but well trimmed.

1. What data deviate from normal findings, suggesting a need for further investigation?

2. What additional questions could be asked by the examiner to clarify symptoms?

3. What additional examination data should be assessed?

4. What type of problem(s) do you think the patient may have?

CLINICAL REASONING

1. A 72-year-old man presents to the clinic with a lesion on his cheek. He says it has been there for years, but his wife has been nagging him to "get it checked out in case it is cancer." After examination, you determine the lesion to be a benign mole. However, you tell the patient to "keep an eye on it." What warning signs would you discuss with him?

2. A mother brings her 3-year-old child to the pediatric clinic, informing the examiner that the child is "red all over and cries frequently." The examiner notes a rash on the child's skin. What specific characteristics should be noted when examining and documenting a skin lesion?

Patient Safety Consideration

While doing a routine physical examination on a young man, you note that his face, ears, neck, chest, upper back, and arms are deeply tanned. What information would help you individualize teaching about safety from ultraviolet (UV) radiation?

CONTENT REVIEW QUESTIONS

Multiple Choice

Circle the best answer for each of the following questions.

1. Milia are an expected finding in which age group?
   a. Newborns
   b. Young children
   c. Adolescents
   d. Older adults

2. An older patient asks the examiner, "Is this spot on my chin a cancer?" Which of the following would indicate a need for further medical investigation?
   a. Reddish-brown color of the lesion
   b. Presence on his chin for 20 years
   c. Bleeds easily when it is touched
   d. Slightly raised and circumscribed

3. A 6-year-old girl has freckles over her nose and cheeks. Freckles are a type of
   a. macule.
   b. papule.
   c. nodule.
   d. petechiae.

4. What grade should be assigned to a pressure ulcer over the coccyx that is open and shallow, showing a red-pink wound bed?
   a. Stage I
   b. Stage II
   c. Stage III
   d. Stage IV

5. Why do some infants develop a yellowish skin tone on the third or fourth day of life?
   a. Increased formation of subcutaneous tissue causes a yellow hue.
   b. Capillaries broken during the birth process turn the skin yellow as bruises heal.
   c. Yellowish color results from increased fat metabolism and heat production.
   d. Red blood cells that hemolyze after birth may cause a yellow skin hue.

6. An adolescent patient asks the examiner why teens have more problems with acne than children. Which of the following would be an appropriate response?
   a. "Children have better hygiene habits than adolescents because of parental guidance."
   b. "Adolescents have reduced blood flow to the epidermal layer of the skin, making them more susceptible to infections."
   c. "At puberty, adolescents begin to secrete more oil from their sebaceous glands."
   d. "Children have very little skin mass, which prevents development of acne."

7. Chloasma is an expected finding in which of the following?
   a. Newborns
   b. Adolescents
   c. Pregnant women
   d. Older adults

8. While examining the skin of an 87-year-old woman, the examiner observes significant tenting. Which of the following age-associated changes best explains this finding?
   a. Small skin tags form on the neck and back.
   b. The skin becomes thin and takes on a parchment-like appearance.
   c. The skin becomes dry, with significant flaking.
   d. There is loss of adipose tissue and loss of elasticity.

9. When assessing for the presence of clubbing, the examiner specifically examines the
   a. width of the nail base.
   b. angle of the nail base.
   c. thickness of the nail.
   d. color of the nail.

10. Which type of lesion sometimes grows out of an already-present nevus?
   a. Malignant melanoma
   b. Squamous cell carcinoma
   c. Basal cell carcinoma
   d. Kaposi sarcoma

11. A skin lesion is described as sessile by the examiner. This means that the lesion
   a. does not have a stalk.
   b. is freely moveable.
   c. bleeds easily.
   d. has a spongy consistency.

12. The examiner notes a large blue-black spot on the buttock of a 4-week-old black neonate. The mother states that the infant was born with it. The examiner should recognize that this
   a. is a common finding.
   b. may indicate child abuse.
   c. is related to birth trauma.
   d. suggests a congenital defect.

13. Which of the following may be associated with neurofibromatosis or pulmonary stenosis?
   a. Café au lait patches
   b. Nevus vasculosus
   c. Port-wine limb stain
   d. Spider angioma

14. Which lesion is an expected finding on the skin of healthy older adults?
   a. Acne vulgaris
   b. Cherry angioma
   c. Miliaria
   d. Trichotillomania

15. When palpating skin surfaces for temperature, the examiner should use the
   a. palmar aspect of the hand.
   b. fingertips of the dominant hand.
   c. dorsal aspect of the hands or fingers.
   d. ulnar surface of the hand.

16. Hyperkeratosis is noted on a patient's palms and soles. The examiner recognizes that this
   a. may be a sign of a systemic disorder.
   b. may be an indication of a congenital heart defect.
   c. is common among individuals with Down syndrome.
   d. is considered a normal finding.

17. A patient with diabetes presents to the clinic complaining of an infected foot. Upon removing the patient's sock, the examiner notes an odor that resembles rotting apples. This finding is consistent with what type of infection?
   a. *Pseudomonas aeruginosa*
   b. Proteus
   c. Viridans streptococci
   d. *Clostridium*

18. Which finding is consistent with a physical abuse injury in a toddler?
   a. Burn to the skin with a splash pattern
   b. Bruising of the skin over soft tissue
   c. Bruising of the skin over a bony prominence
   d. Café au lait patches

19. Which of the following techniques helps the examiner determine whether a palpable skin mass is filled with fluid?
   a. Using a Wood's lamp
   b. Palpating
   c. Transilluminating
   d. Noting the odor of the lesion

20. Which of the following findings suggests that a patient has a fungal infection of the nail beds?
   a. The nail bed is wide and thick.
   b. The nail plate has a central depression, causing a spoon appearance.
   c. Superficial white spots are present in the nail plate.
   d. The nail plate is yellow and crumbling.

10 Lymphatic System

LEARNING OBJECTIVES

After studying Chapter 10 in the textbook and completing this section of the laboratory manual, students should be able to:
1. Conduct a history related to the lymphatic system.
2. Describe techniques for physical examination of the lymphatic system.
3. Identify normal age and condition variations of the lymphatic system.
4. Differentiate normal findings from abnormal findings.
5. Analyze symptoms or clinical findings, relating them to common pathologic conditions.

TERMINOLOGY REVIEW

Check your understanding of terminology related to the lymphatic system. Using the space provided, write the word or phrase from the list next to the appropriate descriptor.

Acute suppurative lymphadenitis	**Lymphangioma**
Fluctuant	**Lymphangitis**
Lymph	**Lymphedema**
Lymphadenitis	**Matted**
Lymphadenopathy	**Shotty nodes**

1. _____: small nontender nodes that feel like BBs or buckshot under the skin.

2. _____: clear, sometimes milky-colored or yellow-tinged fluid containing a variety of white blood cells, most of which are lymphocytes, and an occasional red blood cell.

3. _____: a congenital malformation of dilated lymphatics.

4. _____: infection and inflammation of a lymph node; may affect a single node or localized group of nodes.

5. _____: enlarged lymph nodes.

6. _____: inflammation of the lymphatics that drain an area of infection; tender erythematous streaks extend proximally from the infected area; regional nodes may also be tender.

7. _____: edematous swelling caused by excessive accumulation of lymph fluid in tissues, caused by inadequate lymph drainage.

8. _____: wavelike motion that is felt when the node is palpated.

9. _____: group of nodes that feel connected and seem to move as a unit.

10. _____: inflamed and enlarged lymph node(s).

Anatomy Review

On the illustration below, complete the activities as instructed.

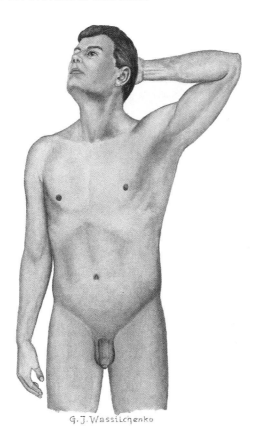

G. J. Wassilchenko

1. Mark the palpable lymph nodes in various regions.

2. Label the various regions of the lymph nodes that you have marked.

3. Indicate with numbers (1 to 6) the order in which you would palpate the head for lymph node examination.

Matching

Match each lymph node with its corresponding location.

Lymph Node	Location
1. Preauricular	a. Behind the tip of the mandible
2. Postauricular	b. Posterior triangle along the edge of the trapezius muscle
3. Occipital	c. Superficial to the mastoid process
4. Submental	d. Halfway between the angle and tip of the mandible
5. Submandibular	e. Above and behind the clavicle
6. Superficial cervical	f. Deep under the sternomastoid muscle
7. Deep cervical	g. Overlying the sternomastoid muscle
8. Posterior cervical	h. Base of the skull
9. Supraclavicular	i. Above and in front of the ear

Clinical Case Study

A 16-year-old male presents with fatigue and weakness. Listed below are data collected by the examiner during an interview and examination.

INTERVIEW DATA

The patient indicates that he keeps a busy schedule with school, basketball, and work. He has always been a good student, but now he seems to be having a harder time keeping up with everything. He feels he is beginning to let his family and friends down because fatigue and weakness are interfering with his performance at school and on the basketball court. He does not want to quit his job because he is saving for college. When asked about other symptoms, he denies changes in appetite or abdominal problems but reports that he thinks he sometimes has a fever.

EXAMINATION DATA

General survey: Alert, thin male. Height, 5 feet 7 inches. Weight, 140 pounds.

Skin: Pink color. No evidence of bruising. No skin discoloration.

Head and neck: Enlarged and firm cervical lymph nodes. Supraclavicular nodes also palpable.

Thorax: Respirations even and unlabored, clear to auscultation. Heart rate and rhythm regular.

Abdomen: Bowel sounds auscultated. Abdomen soft, nontender, and nondistended.

Musculoskeletal: Moves all extremities; symmetric. Moves joints without tenderness.

1. What data deviate from normal findings, suggesting a need for further investigation?

2. What additional questions could be asked by the examiner to clarify symptoms?

3. What additional examination data should be obtained?

4. What type of problem(s) do you think the patient may have?

CLINICAL REASONING

1. How does the lymph system examination of an infant or young child differ from that used for an adult and an older adult? Indicate how findings change with aging.

CONTENT REVIEW QUESTIONS

Multiple Choice

Circle the best answer for each of the following questions.

1. During an examination, which of the following questions would be most appropriate for the examiner to ask a patient to elicit information about the lymph system?
   a. "Are you aware of any lumps?"
   b. "Have you had a change in appetite?"
   c. "Do your lymph nodes hurt?"
   d. "Where are your largest lymph nodes?"

2. While palpating lymph nodes on an adult, the examiner should remember that
   a. tubercular nodes are hot and firm to the touch.
   b. nodes that are fixed and palpable are a normal finding.
   c. heavy pressure is required to locate and identify nodes.
   d. easily palpable nodes are generally not found in healthy adults.

3. In comparison with those of a young adult, the lymph nodes of an older adult will be
   a. large and soft.
   b. small and fatty.
   c. hard and irregular.
   d. large and hard.

4. A 19-year-old man has a severe infection involving the fifth digit of his right hand. Where should the examiner expect to palpate enlarged and tender lymph nodes?
   a. Radial aspect of the right wrist
   b. Palmar aspect of the right hand
   c. Lateral aspect of the right forearm
   d. Medial aspect of the right elbow

5. Which of the following examination findings in an adult is a major cause for concern?
   a. A palpable fluctuant lymph node movable under the examiner's fingers.
   b. A palpable hard lymph node fixed in its setting.
   c. A palpable soft lymph node approximately 2 mm in size.
   d. Absence of any palpable lymph nodes.

6. The most common causes of acute suppurative lymphadenitis are which organisms?
   a. *Pseudomonas* and *Clostridium* spp.
   b. *Streptococcus* and *Staphylococcus* spp.
   c. *Candida* and *Chlamydia* spp.
   d. A*spergillus* and *Escherichia* spp.

7. The examiner typically assesses the lymph system using which of the following methods?
   a. Assesses the entire lymph system as a unit, exploring all accessible nodes.
   b. Assesses both the superficial and deep nodes using palpation and a Doppler study.
   c. Assesses the lymph system region by region as each body system is assessed.
   d. Assesses the lymph nodes only when the patient's history suggests a need to do so.

8. A 2-month-old infant is brought to the clinic for immunizations. The examiner palpates enlarged inguinal nodes. What additional finding might explain the enlarged nodes?
   a. The mother reports that the infant has colic.
   b. The infant's length and weight are above the 85th percentile.
   c. The infant has a severe diaper rash.
   d. A port-wine stain is present on the infant's left thigh.

9. As the examiner palpates an enlarged lymph node, the patient complains of pain. This is suggestive of
   a. an inflammatory process.
   b. Hodgkin disease.
   c. immature lymph node development.
   d. toxoplasmosis.

10. Which examination method is used to differentiate an enlarged lymph node from a cyst?
    a. Palpation
    b. Auscultation
    c. Biopsy
    d. Transillumination

11. Which of the following methods best describes how to assess supraclavicular lymph nodes?
    a. Have the patient assume a supine position and then hold his or her breath.
    b. Place the patient in the Trendelenburg position and illuminate the lymph nodes with a bright light.
    c. Palpate deeply behind the clavicles as the patient takes a deep breath.
    d. Hook fingers over the clavicles with the patient in a sitting position, with head flexed.

12. The examiner notes enlarged tonsils in a young child. The examiner should recognize that this
    a. is an indication of a retropharyngeal abscess.
    b. may be an early indication of Epstein-Barr virus.
    c. is an indication that the child has lymphoma.
    d. may be a normal finding.

13. In addition to the head, neck, axillae, and inguinal area, the examiner may also assess lymph nodes in which location?
    a. On the palmar aspect of the hands
    b. In the popliteal region
    c. In the patellar region
    d. On the dorsum of the foot

14. Which of the following is an assessment technique that can differentiate mumps from cervical adenitis?
    a. Palpating for the angle of the jaw
    b. Palpating enlarged lymph nodes
    c. Noting painful lymph nodes
    d. Noting swelling of the face

15. On examining a patient, you find matted occipital lymph nodes. What do you do to facilitate subsequent assessment for change in the matted nodes?
    a. Outline the mass with a skin pen.
    b. Tattoo the center of the mass.
    c. Mark 12, 3, 6, and 9 o'clock positions on the periphery of the mass with a skin pencil.
    d. Use calipers to obtain the diameter of the mass.

16. A patient presents to the office with a complaint of a lump in the neck. What would you expect to feel if the problem involved a cancer that had spread through the lymph system?
    a. A soft lymph node less than 0.5 cm in size
    b. Multiple small, hard, nontender nodes
    c. A single, firm node affixed to underlying tissue
    d. Solitary, tender, matted node of variable size

17. Normal cervical lymph nodes typically are
    a. matted.
    b. tender to palpation.
    c. rubbery.
    d. smaller than 1 cm.

18. On examination of a patient, you palpate enlarged preauricular and submandibular lymph nodes. Which term can be used to describe this finding?
    a. Lymphadenopathy
    b. Lymphadenitis
    c. Lymphangitis
    d. Lymphedema

19. How should the patient be positioned when you palpate for left inguinal lymph nodes?
    a. Standing, with weight on the right leg
    b. Sitting, with the legs dangling
    c. Supine, with knees slightly bent
    d. Supine, with the left leg externally rotated

20. Which finding is the most concerning?
    a. 3-mm occipital lymph node in a neonate
    b. 6-mm postauricular lymph node in a 1 year old
    c. 0.5-cm cervical lymph node in a 3 year old
    d. 0.8-cm supraclavicular lymph node in a 5 year old

11 Head and Neck

LEARNING OBJECTIVES

After studying Chapter 11 in the textbook and completing this section of the laboratory manual, students should be able to:
1. Conduct a history related to the head and neck.
2. Discuss examination techniques for the head and neck.
3. Identify normal age and condition variations related to the head and neck.
4. Recognize findings that deviate from expected findings.
5. Relate symptoms and clinical findings to common pathologic conditions.

TERMINOLOGY REVIEW

Check your understanding of terminology related to the head and neck. Using the space provided, write the word or phrase from the list next to the appropriate descriptor.

Bruit	Mastoid fontanel
Bulging fontanel	Microcephaly
Chloasma	Molding
Craniosynostosis	Ossification
Encephalocele	Plagiocephaly
Exophthalmos	Tic
Facies	Torticollis
Macewen sign	Webbing

1. _____: a third (abnormal) fontanel located between the anterior and posterior fontanels; common in individuals with Down syndrome.

2. _____: facial discoloration common during pregnancy; also called the mask of pregnancy; this fades after delivery.

3. _____: distortion in the shape of a baby's skull, most often positional in origin; also called flat head syndrome.

4. _____: general appearance of the space and features of the head and neck that, when considered together, are characteristics of a clinical condition or syndrome.

5. _____: excessive posterior cervical skin or an unusually short neck, usually associated with chromosomal anomalies.

6. _____: a condition in which the fontanel feels tense and protrudes above the level of the skull bones when the child is sitting.

7. _____: a condition in which the circumference of the head is smaller than normal; associated with intellectual disability and failure of the brain to develop normally.

8. _____: a soft, rushing sound that may be detected in the hypervascular thyroid.

9. _____: a condition in which the neck is twisted secondary to excessive contraction of the sternocleidomastoid muscle (also called "wry neck"); often the result of birth trauma or intrauterine malposition; acquired torticollis may be caused by tumor, trauma, palsy of cranial nerve IV, muscle spasm, infection, or drug ingestion.

10. _____: a neural tube defect with protrusions of brain and membranes that cover it through openings in the skull; has a genetic component often occurring in families with history of spina bifida or anencephaly.

11. _____: an abnormal shaping of the infant's head caused by the shifting and overlapping of bones during vaginal delivery.

12. _____: bone tissue formation; begins in sutures after brain growth is completed at about 6 years of age.

13. _____: a condition that results from the premature closing of sutures before brain growth is complete; leads to a misshapen skull that is not accompanied by mental retardation.

14. _____: increased prominence of the eyes.

15. _____: percussion of the skull near the junction of the frontal, temporal, and parietal bones will be resonant; the sign associated with increased intracranial pressure after fontanels are closed.

16. _____: a spasmodic contraction of the face, head, or neck.

APPLICATION TO CLINICAL PRACTICE

Matching

Match each type of headache with its corresponding characteristic.

Type of Headache	Characteristic
_____ 1. Hypertensive headache	a. May be brought on by extreme anger.
_____ 2. Migraine headache	b. May be brought on by alcohol consumption.
_____ 3. Muscular tension headache	c. More common in females.
_____ 4. Headache from temporal arteritis	d. Begins in morning and decreases as day progresses.
_____ 5. Cluster headache	e. Age of onset typically older adult.

Identify the structures of the neck labeled on the illustration. Using the list of terms below the illustration, write the correct term in the blank next to the corresponding letter. Use each term once.

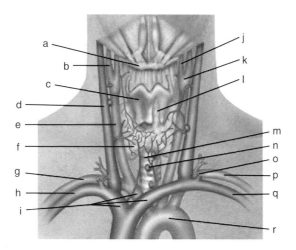

a. _____	External carotid artery
b. _____	Lymph node
c. _____	Carotid sinus
d. _____	Thyroid gland
e. _____	Hyoid bone
f. _____	Trachea
g. _____	External jugular vein
h. _____	Internal jugular vein
i. _____	Right subclavian artery
j. _____	Brachiocephalic artery and vein
k. _____	Internal carotid artery
l. _____	Common carotid artery
m. _____	Pyramidal lobe (thyroid gland)
n. _____	Arch of aorta
o. _____	Left subclavian vein
p. _____	Left subclavian artery
q. _____	Right subclavian vein
r. _____	Thyroid cartilage

Concepts Application

Complete the table below by listing the common characteristics of the physical appearance and demeanor of a patient with hyperthyroidism and a patient with hypothyroidism.

System or Structure	Hyperthyroidism	Hypothyroidism
Weight		
Emotional state		
Temperature preference		
Hair		
Skin		
Neck		
Gastrointestinal		
Eyes		

Case Study

A 44-year-old carpenter comes to the emergency department because of a severe headache. Listed below are data collected by the examiner.

INTERVIEW DATA

When the examiner attempts to ask the patient about the headache, he cries out, "I can't take this anymore! It hurts too much!" His wife says that her husband has been getting these headaches a couple of times a day for the past week now—sometimes at night—so he has not been sleeping well. She also indicates that he had headaches like these about a year ago and that they lasted about a month. When the examiner asks the patient whether he experiences nausea or sensitivity to light, he replies, "No, I just get a stuffy nose." His wife says that he is constantly worried about whether—and when—the headache will come back because, as she says, "We don't know what is causing them, and nothing seems to help them go away." She says that he feels like all he can do is hold his head and pray that the pain will stop.

EXAMINATION DATA

General survey: Alert, well-nourished man of average weight, in moderate distress. He is unable to lie still and paces the floor around the examination area, holding the left side of his head (over his eye and forehead).

Head and neck: Skull is intact, with no lumps, depressions, or tenderness. No abnormalities are found with facial structures. The head is centered on the neck; the trachea is midline. Thyroid is in midline position and of normal size.

1. What data deviate from normal findings, suggesting a need for further investigation?

2. What additional questions could be asked by the examiner to clarify symptoms?

3. What additional examination data should be obtained?

CLINICAL REASONING

1. What role does the technique of percussion play in the examination of the head and neck?

2. What role does the technique of auscultation play in the examination of the head and neck?

Patient Safety Consideration

The mother of a neonate says that she doesn't want to put her baby on his back to sleep because she doesn't want his head to be malformed. How do you reply?

CONTENT REVIEW QUESTIONS

Multiple Choice

Circle the best answer for each of the following questions:

1. In which group is a slight enlargement of the thyroid gland detected on ultrasound considered a normal finding?
   a. Infants
   b. Adolescents
   c. Pregnant women
   d. Native Americans or American Indians

2. Which of the following questions is most appropriate to ask a female patient with a suspected thyroid problem?
   a. "How much alcohol do you drink?"
   b. "Have you noticed a change in your sleep pattern or energy level?"
   c. "Do you have headaches?"
   d. "Are you currently menstruating?"

3. An infant with an alcoholic mother is admitted to the hospital with fetal alcohol syndrome. What assessment finding is consistent with this syndrome?
   a. Ear dysplasia
   b. Moon face
   c. Torticollis
   d. Thin upper lip

4. Which of the following findings in an older patient would be considered a normal consequence of aging?
   a. Narrowed palpebral fissures
   b. Pulsating fontanels
   c. Uneven movement of the tongue
   d. Fibrosis of the thyroid gland

5. Assessment of an infant's fontanels is best performed while the infant is
   a. calm and in an upright position.
   b. sleeping in a lateral position.
   c. supine and awake.
   d. held at a 45-degree angle.

6. What problem is suggested by a positive Cardarelli sign?
   a. Ocular migraine
   b. Aortic aneurysm
   c. Hashimoto disease
   d. Thyroid cyst

7. A 6-month-old infant is brought to the clinic for immunizations. While examining the baby, the examiner notes that the anterior fontanel has not closed. What is the significance of this finding?
   a. This indicates a slight developmental delay.
   b. There may be a nutritional deficiency.
   c. This finding is consistent with hydrocephaly.
   d. This is a normal finding.

8. Preterm infants often have
   a. long, narrow heads.
   b. broad nose bridges.
   c. low-set ears.
   d. webbed necks.

9. The presence of a nodular thyroid is a normal finding in
   a. infants.
   b. adolescents.
   c. pregnant women.
   d. older adults.

10. Webbing, excessive posterior cervical skin, and a short neck are signs associated with
    a. Asian heritage.
    b. chromosomal anomalies.
    c. Cushing syndrome.
    d. malnutrition.

11. Transillumination of the skull should be performed
    a. in infants of mothers with diabetes.
    b. in infants with a history of traumatic birth.
    c. when an infant has a facial nerve palsy.
    d. in infants with suspected intracranial lesions.

12. Which of the following findings suggests an inflammation of the thyroid gland?
    a. Gritty sensation when the thyroid is palpated
    b. Movement of the thyroid when the patient swallows
    c. Vertical ridges palpated on the thyroid gland
    d. Swollen and red skin overlying the thyroid gland

13. A patient demonstrates asymmetry of the mouth. The examiner suspects a problem with the
    a. inferior facial nerve.
    b. thyroid gland.
    c. peripheral trigeminal nerve.
    d. salivary duct.

14. A patient presents with complaints of throbbing, unilateral head pain associated with nausea and vomiting. Which problem is suggested by these symptoms?
    a. Temporal arteritis.
    b. Cluster headache.
    c. Subarachnoid hemorrhage.
    d. Migraine headache.

15. You are palpating a thyroid gland and note that it is enlarged bilaterally. What is your next step in the examination process?
    a. Listen for vascular sounds over the thyroid lobes.
    b. Examine the patient for enlarged lymph nodes.
    c. Check for a deviated trachea.
    d. Listen for a bruit over the carotids.

12 Eyes

LEARNING OBJECTIVES

After studying Chapter 12 in the textbook and completing this section of the laboratory manual, students should be able to:
1. Conduct a history related to the eyes and vision.
2. Discuss examination techniques for the eyes.
3. Identify normal age and condition variations related to the eyes.
4. Recognize findings that deviate from expected findings.
5. Relate symptoms or clinical findings to common pathologic conditions.

TERMINOLOGY REVIEW

Check your understanding of terminology related to the assessment of the eyes. Using the space provided, write the word or phrase from the list next to the appropriate descriptor.

Adie pupil (tonic pupil)   Lipemia retinalis
Anisocoria   Miosis
Argyll Robertson pupil   Mydriasis
Band keratopathy   Nystagmus
Cotton wool spot   Papilledema
Drusen bodies   Presbyopia
Ectropion   Pterygium
Entropion   Ptosis
Glaucomatous optic nerve cupping Red reflex
Hemianopia   Strabismus
Hordeolum   Xanthelasma
Hypertelorism

1. _____: progressive weakening of accommodation (focusing power); the major physiologic change that occurs after the age of 45 years.

2. _____: eyelid, usually lower, turned outward away from the eye.

3. _____: a creamy-white appearance of retinal vessels that occurs when the serum triglyceride level exceeds 2000 mg/dL of blood.

4. _____: abnormal growth of conjunctiva that extends over the cornea from the limbus; occurs more commonly on the nasal side.

5. _____: unequal pupillary size, more prominent in darkness, may be congenital.

6. _____: small, discrete yellow spots on the retina.

7. _____: physiologic disc margins that are raised, with a lowered central area.

8. _____: deposition of calcium in the superficial cornea.

9. _____: defective vision in half of the visual field.

10. _____: drooping of the upper eyelid; indicates a congenital or acquired weakness of the levator muscle or a paresis of a branch of the third cranial nerve.

11. _____: an acute suppurative inflammation of the follicle of an eyelash that can lead to an erythematous or yellow lump or sty caused by staphylococcal organisms.

12. _____: pupil that is dilated and reacts slowly or fails to react to light; responds to convergence, caused by impairment of postganglionic parasympathetic innervation.

13. _____: condition characterized by elevated plaque of cholesterol; commonly found on the nasal portion of the upper or lower eyelid.

14. _____: eyelid, usually lower, turned inward, resulting in corneal and conjunctival irritation with an increased risk of secondary infection.

15. _____: involuntary rhythmic movement of the eyes that can occur in a horizontal, vertical, rotary, or mixed pattern.

16. _____: condition in which both eyes do not focus on the same object simultaneously, although either eye can focus independently.

17. _____: bilateral, miotic, irregularly shaped pupils that fail to constrict with light but retain constriction with convergence.

18. _____: ill-defined yellow areas caused by infarction of nerve layer of the retina.

19. _____: eyes widely spaced apart; may be associated with craniofacial defects, including some with intellectual disability.

20. _____: loss of definition of the optic disc; initially occurs superiorly and inferiorly and then nasally and temporally central vessels are pushed forward.

21. _____: pupillary constriction, usually less than 2 mm in diameter.

22. _____: pupillary dilation, usually more than 6 mm in diameter.

23. _____: response caused by light illuminating the retina.

APPLICATION TO CLINICAL PRACTICE

Matching 1

Match each clinical finding with its corresponding associated factor.

Clinical Finding	Associated Factor
____ 1. Adie pupil	a. Uremia
____ 2. Anisocoria	b. Congenital finding in 20% of normal population
____ 3. Argyll Robertson pupil	c. Diabetic neuropathy or alcoholism
____ 4. Mydriasis	d. Oculomotor nerve damage
____ 5. Eye deviated laterally, downward	e. Neurosyphilis or midbrain lesion
____ 6. Corneal arcus	f. Lipid deposition

61

In the left-hand column below, list the structures included in the external examination of the eye in the order in which they should be assessed. To the right of each structure, identify what specifically should be examined.

Structure	What Should Be Examined
1.	
2.	
3.	
4.	
5.	
6.	
7.	

Concepts Application 2

Referring to the following illustration, describe the position of the lesion based on disc diameter.

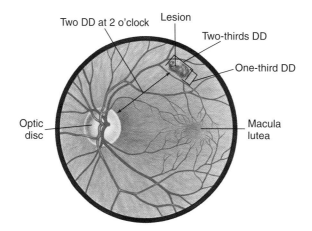

1. a. Location

   b. Length

   c. Width

Matching 2

Match each examination finding with its corresponding diagnosis.

Examination Finding	Diagnosis
____ 1. Opacity in the lens	a. Lipemia retinalis
____ 2. Microaneurysms	b. Glaucoma
____ 3. Eye vessels becoming progressively pink and then white as triglyceride levels rise	c. Cataract
____ 4. Characteristic appearance of the optic nerve—increased cupping	d. Background diabetic retinopathy
____ 5. Ill-defined mass arising from the retina in children	e. Retinoblastoma

Case Study

A 32-year-old single white male with insulin-dependent diabetes mellitus seeks care for a vision problem. Listed below are data collected during an interview and examination.

INTERVIEW DATA

Although the patient has been compliant with his treatment regimen, he has had poor control of his diabetes. He presents to the clinic with complaints of significant reduction in vision over the past couple of weeks. He tells the nurse, "I can't lose my vision because I won't be able to keep my job. If I can't see, I don't know how I will take care of my diabetes or how I will maintain my income."

EXAMINATION DATA

General survey: Anxious, well-nourished male.

Eyes: Snellen test—left eye, 20/70; right eye, 20/70 +2; Both eyes, 20/60 +1; reduced peripheral vision. Normal extraocular movement and corneal light reflex. Eyelids and eyelashes symmetric. Conjunctiva clear bilaterally. Sclera is white; corneas clear. Lacrimal structures without tearing. Pupils are equal and round and react to light.

Internal eye examination: Retinal vessels hemorrhagic. New vessels present. Findings consistent with proliferative diabetic retinopathy.

1. What data deviate from normal findings, suggesting a need for further investigation?

2. What additional questions could the examiner ask to clarify symptoms?

3. What previous examination findings should be considered if available?

4. What problem(s) does this patient have?

CLINICAL REASONING

1. A 5-year-old child is brought in for a routine physical examination. Describe what components of the eye examination are appropriate for a child of this age without specific eye or visual complaints.

2. While examining the eye, the examiner notes retinal vessels. How are arteries and veins differentiated?

Patient Safety Consideration

1. Would you administer a mydriatic agent to dilate the pupils of a pregnant patient?

2. How would you identify patients at risk for acute-angle glaucoma from instillation of a mydriatic?

CONTENT REVIEW QUESTIONS

Multiple Choice

Circle the best answer for each of the following questions:

1. Which of the following is relevant information for a history and examination of a child's eyes and vision?
   a. Immunization history
   b. Growth milestones
   c. Birth weight
   d. Academic performance

2. Before instilling a mydriatic eyedrop, the examiner should
   a. assess the corneal reflex.
   b. observe the limbus while shining focused light tangentially.
   c. assess intraocular pressure.
   d. observe the eye for vascular changes.

3. The examiner screens a 5-year-old child for nystagmus during which part of the eye examination?
   a. Assessment of visual acuity
   b. Inspection of the macula of the eye with an ophthalmoscope
   c. Checking movement of the eyes through the six cardinal fields of gaze
   d. Palpation of the eyelids and orbit

4. Which of the following correctly describes the method used to assess accommodation?
   a. Shine a light into the pupil; note constriction.
   b. Note pupil constriction as gaze shifts from across the room to an object about 4 inches away.
   c. Note ocular movement as the patient follows an object through the six cardinal fields.
   d. Cover one eye of the patient with a card; then remove the card, noting any deviation from a fixed gaze.

5. Which of the following should be used to test for near vision?
   a. Rosenbaum chart
   b. Amsler grid
   c. Confrontation test
   d. Cover–uncover test

6. To visualize the macula, the examiner should ask the patient to
   a. blink the eye several times quickly.
   b. lie in a supine position.
   c. look directly into the light of the ophthalmoscope.
   d. direct his or her eye gaze on an object to the left and then to the right.

7. Which of the following is considered a routine part of a newborn examination?
   a. Assessing red reflex
   b. Assessing extraocular movements with six fields of gaze
   c. Funduscopic examination
   d. Visual acuity

8. Which examination finding may be indicative of a retro-orbital tumor?
   a. Episcleritis
   b. Argyll Robertson pupil
   c. Unilateral exophthalmos
   d. Retinitis pigmentosa

9. A patient tells the examiner, "I have a loss of vision in the outer half of each eye." Which of the following underlying problems should the examiner consider?
   a. Diabetes
   b. Pituitary tumor
   c. Glaucoma
   d. Cytomegalovirus infection

10. Which of the following would be asked about as part of a family history?
    a. Eye dominance
    b. Pupil size
    c. Retinoblastoma
    d. Sty

11. A patient has vision that, at best, is 20/210. This patient is considered
    a. legally blind.
    b. mildly myopic.
    c. moderately hyperopic.
    d. unilaterally anisocoric.

12. Which of the following is the correct technique for performing an ophthalmoscopic examination? Examine the patient's
    a. right eye with your right eye and the left eye with your left eye.
    b. right eye with your left eye and the left eye with your right eye.
    c. right and left eyes with your dominant eye.
    d. right and left eyes with your nondominant eye.

13. Failure to elicit a red reflex in a young child may indicate
    a. congenital glaucoma.
    b. myosis.
    c. retinopathy.
    d. retinoblastoma.

14. An examiner is most likely to observe pseudostrabismus in which of the following groups?
    a. Older adults with ectropions
    b. Infants with epicanthal folds
    c. Pregnant women with cloasma
    d. Children with ptosis

15. A cobblestone appearance of the conjunctiva is most likely related to
    a. subconjunctival hemorrhage.
    b. allergic or infectious conjunctivitis.
    c. lagophthalmos.
    d. cytomegalovirus infection.

16. On examining the eyes of a 48-year-old patient, you note peripheral fundus changes and vessels that appear whitish. The most likely cause for these findings is
    a. floaters.
    b. lipemia retinalis.
    c. hypertension.
    d. glaucomatous optic nerve cupping.

17. Which of the following cranial nerves innervate the six muscles that control eye movement?
    a. II, III, IV
    b. III, IV, V
    c. III, IV, VI
    d. IV, V, VI

18. When you are examining the eyelid, you note ptosis on the right side. Which cranial nerve innervates the muscle that elevates the upper eyelid?
    a. CN II
    b. CN III
    c. CN IV
    d. CN VI

19. During the eye examination of a 57-year-old patient you note that his pupils are not equal in size; however, they react to light and accommodation. This is called
    a. anisocoria.
    b. Adie pupil.
    c. Hirschberg test.
    d. amblyopia.

20. Which is the cause of proliferative diabetic retinopathy?
    a. Fluctuating blood glucose levels
    b. Excessive intraocular pressure
    c. Deposition of calcium
    d. Anoxic stimulation

Ears, Nose, and Throat

After studying Chapter 13 in the textbook and completing this section of the laboratory manual, students should be able to:
1. Conduct a history related to the ears, nose, and throat.
2. Discuss examination techniques for the ears, nose, and throat.
3. Identify normal age and condition variations related to the ears, nose, and throat.
4. Recognize findings that deviate from expected findings.
5. Relate symptoms and clinical findings to common pathologic conditions.

TERMINOLOGY REVIEW

Check your understanding of terminology related to the assessment of the ears, nose, and throat. Using the space provided, write the word or phrase from the list next to the appropriate descriptor.

Cerumen	Otosclerosis
Cheilitis	Presbycusis
Conductive hearing loss	Rinne test
Epistaxis	Sensorineural hearing loss
Epstein pearls	Torus
Fordyce spots	Vertigo
Frenulum	Weber test
Ossicles	Xerostomia

1. _____: hearing test that compares bone conduction of sound with air conduction of sound.

2. _____: small fold of tissue that attaches at a midway point between the ventral surface of the tongue and the tip and attaches the tongue to the floor of the mouth.

3. _____: dry mouth.

4. _____: bone deposition immobilizing the stapes.

5. _____: hearing loss resulting from reduced transmission of sound to the middle ear; may result from an excess deposition of bone cells along the ossicle chain, causing fixation of the stapes in the oval window, cerumen impaction, or a sclerotic tympanic membrane.

6. _____: earwax, secreted by the apocrine glands in the distal third of the ear canal; provides an acidic pH environment that inhibits the growth of microorganisms; comes in two types—wet and dry; type is a genetic trait.

7. _____: a screening test for hearing that tests the lateralization of sound.

8. _____: bumps that may appear on the buccal mucosa and lips; ectopic sebaceous glands that appear as small, yellow-white raised lesions.

9. _____: hearing impairment that results from a disorder of the inner ear, damage to cranial nerve VIII, or damage to the brain.

10. _____: small whitish-yellow masses at the juncture between the hard and soft palate.

11. _____: bony protuberance on the midline of the hard palate.

12. _____: the three small bones of the inner ear known as the malleus, incus, and stapes that transmit sound from the tympanic membrane to the oval window to the inner ear.

13. _____: dry, cracked lips; may be caused by dehydration from wind chapping, dentures, braces, or excessive lip licking.

14. _____: nosebleed.

15. _____: bilateral sensorineural hearing loss associated with aging resulting from changes in the inner ear or vestibular nerve.

16. _____: the illusion of rotational movement experienced by a patient; often caused by a disorder of the inner ear.

APPLICATION TO CLINICAL PRACTICE

Matching
Match each clinical finding with its corresponding associated factors.

Clinical Finding	Associated Factors
_____ 1. Ménière disease	a. Dry mouth
_____ 2. Sinusitis	b. Headache, nasal discharge, infection of one or more of the paranasal sinuses
_____ 3. Peritonsillar abscess	c. Ear fullness, tinnitus, vertigo' hearing loss
_____ 4. Xerostomia	d. Dysphagia, fever, fetid breath, referred pain to the ears
_____ 5. Presbycusis	e. Conductive hearing loss resulting from bony overgrowth of the stapes
_____ 6. Otitis externa	f. Epithelial growth that migrates through a perforation in the tympanic membrane
_____ 7. Middle ear effusion	g. Bilateral sensorineural hearing loss associated with aging
_____ 8. Cholesteatoma	h. Inflammation of the middle ear resulting in a collection of serous mucoid or purulent fluid
_____ 9. Otosclerosis	i. Infection of the auditory canal

Identify the structures of the middle ear labeled on the illustration below. Using the list of terms provided, write the correct term in the blank next to the corresponding letter. Use each term once.

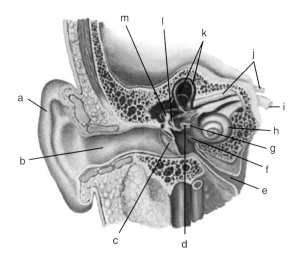

a. _____	Cochlea
b. _____	Malleus
c. _____	Cochlear and vestibular branches of the auditory nerve
d. _____	Round window
e. _____	Stapes and footplate
f. _____	Auricle
g. _____	Semicircular canals
h. _____	External auditory canal
i. _____	Eustachian tube
j. _____	Oval window
k. _____	Incus
l. _____	Facial nerve
m. _____	Tympanic membrane

CLINICAL APPLICATION

Fill in the blanks in the following statements, selecting the appropriate terms from the list below.

Darwin tubercle   Koplik spots

Epstein pearls   malocclusion

1. _____ are white specks with a red base found on the buccal mucosa opposite the first and second molars and may occur in a child with a fever or with rubeola.

2. A _____ appears as a blunt point projecting up from the upper part of the helix of the ear.

3. Improper position of the teeth is referred to as _____.

4. On the roof of the mouth of an infant, _____ appear as small, whitish masses and are considered a normal finding.

Case Study

A 5-year-old Native American girl was brought to the clinic by her mother. Listed below are data collected by the examiner during an interview and examination.

INTERVIEW DATA

The mother tells the examiner that her daughter "has been complaining of ear pain. She has been very hot and crying frequently." She adds, "I wanted to bring her to the clinic yesterday, but my grandmother told me I shouldn't." The mother continues, telling the examiner, "She has been treated many times for this problem over the past several years by the medicine man. Last night, I saw drainage from her ears. Grandmother told me this was a sign that the illness was being chased from the body. I did not know what it was, but I felt scared." The mother indicates that her daughter knows English but that she has never really talked very much.

EXAMINATION DATA

General survey: Small-for-age 5-year-old girl; quiet, flat affect. Does not look at the examiner; does not interact with the mother or the examiner.

External ear examination: Typical position of ears bilaterally. Left ear pinna red. Dried bloody drainage noted on left external ear and in left external canal. Cries when the left ear is touched. Right ear unremarkable.

Internal canal and tympanic membrane: Dried drainage noted in the left ear canal. Tympanic membrane perforated. Right ear tympanic membrane pearly gray; landmarks and light reflex present.

Hearing examination: Whisper test in right ear = correctly repeats four of five words; whisper test in left ear = none of five words repeated. Weber test = hears tuning fork in right ear.

1. What data deviate from normal findings, suggesting a need for further investigation?

2. What additional questions could the examiner ask to clarify symptoms?

3. What additional physical examination, if any, should the examiner complete?

4. What primary problems does the patient have?

CLINICAL REASONING

1. A mother brings her 6-month-old infant to the clinic and tells the examiner, "She has had a fever all night and has been crying for the past hour." The examiner looks in the baby's ears and notes that the tympanic membrane is red. How can the examiner differentiate redness caused by otitis media from redness caused by crying?

Patient Safety Consideration

A 10-year-old patient is brought to the clinic because of decreased hearing in the right ear. On examination, the ear is found to be impacted with cerumen. Your options for managing the problem are to remove the cerumen by irrigating with water or to remove it by using a cerumen spoon. What basic facts do you consider in making this decision?

CONTENT REVIEW QUESTIONS

Multiple Choice

Circle the best answer for each of the following questions.

1. When performing a Weber test, which of the following is considered a normal finding? The patient
   a. hears the tone equally in both ears.
   b. hears the tone better in one ear than in the other.
   c. hears sounds longer when conducted through air than when conducted through bone.
   d. is able to detect tones of varying frequencies and pitches from a tuning fork.

2. Which of the following best explains why infants and toddlers are at greater risk for ear infections than are older children and adults?
   a. Poorly developed immune system
   b. Immature tympanic membrane
   c. Wider, shorter, and more horizontal eustachian tubes
   d. Excess deposition of bone cells along the ossicle

3. Which finding is most likely to suggest a foreign object in the nose of a young child?
   a. The mother states that the child plays with toys.
   b. The examiner notes a purulent discharge from the right side of the child's nose.
   c. The child has a foul-smelling odor from the nose.
   d. The child cries when lying down.

4. The examiner observes a blackish lesion on the top surface of the tongue of an adult patient. The patient indicates that his tongue is painful. Which question by the examiner would be helpful in explaining this finding?
   a. "Have you been taking antibiotics lately?"
   b. "Have you injured your tongue?"
   c. "Have you been diagnosed with mouth cancer before?"
   d. "When was the last time you brushed your teeth?"

5. How would you manipulate the auricle of an older adult patient to ensure maximum visibility of the tympanic membrane through the otoscope?
   a. Pull the auricle down and forward.
   b. Pull the auricle down and back.
   c. Pull the auricle up and forward.
   d. Pull the auricle up and back,

6. The examiner notes that a patient's tonsils are enlarged and that they nearly touch the uvula. This is documented as
   a. 1 + .
   b. 2 + .
   c. 3 + .
   d. 4 + .

7. Which of the following statements made by a 72-year-old patient would indicate a normal process of aging?
   a. "My tongue feels swollen."
   b. "My tonsils are large and sore."
   c. "Food does not taste the same as it used to."
   d. "I have white and black spots under my tongue."

8. Which of the following behaviors, as described by a parent, is most likely to indicate a hearing problem?
   a. "My 4-month-old baby does not seem to respond to loud noises."
   b. "My 5-month-old baby is babbling, but she is not yet saying any words."
   c. "When my 15-month-old baby is talking, I sometimes have a hard time understanding her."
   d. "Sometimes my 3-year-old does not pay attention to me."

9. Which assessment would **not** be included as part of the ENT examination of a 5-year-old child?
   a. Inspection of the teeth
   b. Palpation of frontal sinuses
   c. Elicitation of the gag reflex
   d. Whispered voice hearing evaluation

10. While examining the ear of a 6-week-old infant, the examiner observes a tympanic membrane lacking conical appearance and with a diffuse light reflex. These findings
    a. suggest a congenital abnormality.
    b. suggest a ruptured tympanic membrane.
    c. are classic findings for otitis media in a neonate.
    d. are normal.

11. Rhinorrhea, red and swollen nasal mucosa, nose-bleeds, mucosal scabs, and septum perforation are signs of
    a. chronic allergies.
    b. cocaine abuse.
    c. fungal infection.
    d. turbinate hypertrophy.

12. Which direction do you give to the patient when you are ready to assess the movement of the soft palate?
    a. "Swallow."
    b. "Say ah."
    c. "Breathe through your mouth."
    d. "Stick out your tongue."

13. Clinical signs of sinusitis in adults include which of the following?
    a. Persistent cough, temporal headache, fever over 100°F.
    b. Poor response to decongestants, postnasal drip, previous tonsillectomy.
    c. Purulent nasal discharge, mandibular toothache, nasal allergies.
    d. Maxillary toothache, purulent nasal drainage, persistent cough.

14. What conclusion can you draw when you observe a patient's uvula deviating to the left?
    a. The patient's dominant side is the right.
    b. The patient's dominant side is the left.
    c. There is a problem on the right side.
    d. There is a problem on the left side.

15. When the patient extends his tongue, it deviates to the right. What meaning do you assign to this observation?
    a. The hypoglossal nerve is impaired.
    b. The patient has had a minor stroke.
    c. The frenulum is abnormally short.
    d. The patient has a retropharyngeal abscess.

14 Chest and Lungs

LEARNING OBJECTIVES

After studying Chapter 14 in the textbook and completing this section of the laboratory manual, students should be able to:

1. Describe anatomy and physiology of the chest and lungs.
2. Organize interview questions pertinent to chest and lung examination.
3. Describe appropriate equipment used for chest and lung examination.
4. Relate inspection, palpation, percussion, and auscultation examination techniques to the chest and lungs.
5. Distinguish variations in the health history and physical examination among infants, adolescents, pregnant women, and older adults.
6. Analyze normal examination findings, relating them to examination findings associated with various conditions of the chest and lungs.

TERMINOLOGY REVIEW

Check your understanding of terminology related to the chest and lungs. Using the space provided, write the word or phrase from the list next to the appropriate descriptor.

Apnea	Kussmaul breathing
Biot respirations	Medium crackles
Bronchophony	Pectoriloquy
Bronchovesicular breath sounds	Pleural friction rub
Cheyne-Stokes respiration	Rhonchi
Coarse crackles	Stridor
Crackles	Tracheomalacia
Egophony	Vesicular breath sounds
Fine crackles	Vocal resonance
Hamman sign	Wheeze

1. _____: (sibilant wheeze) musical noise sounding similar to a squeak; most often heard continuously during inspiration or expiration; usually louder during expiration.

2. _____: increased clarity and loudness of spoken sound.

3. _____: a whisper can be clearly heard through the stethoscope; associated with consolidation of lungs.

4. _____: a regular periodic pattern of breathing, with intervals of apnea followed by a crescendo–decrescendo sequence of respirations; often associated with serious illnesses.

5. _____: sound of the spoken word as transmitted through the lung fields; usually muffled and indistinct in quality.

6. _____: high-pitched, piercing sound most often heard during inspiration; it is the result of an obstruction high in the respiratory tree.

7. _____: absence of spontaneous respiration; it may have its origin in the respiratory system or a variety of central nervous system and cardiac abnormalities.

8. _____: high-pitched, discrete, discontinuous crackling sounds heard during the end of inspiration not cleared by a cough.

9. _____: typically moderate in pitch and intensity; heard over major bronchi.

10. _____: deep and usually rapid respirations; the eponym applied to the respiratory effort associated with metabolic acidosis.

11. _____: irregular respirations varying in depth and interrupted by intervals of apnea but lacking repetitive pattern; associated with increased intracranial pressure, respiratory compromise, or brain damage at the level of the medulla.

12. _____: sonorous wheezes; loud, low, course sounds similar to a snore; most often heard continuously during inspiration or expiration.

13. _____: abnormal lung sounds, more often heard on inspiration; characterized by discrete discontinuous sounds; also called rales.

14. _____: a "floppiness" or lack of rigidity of the trachea or airway.

15. _____: greater clarity and increased loudness of spoken words.

16. _____: loud, bubbly noise heard during inspiration not cleared by a cough.

17. _____: mediastinal crunch; found with mediastinal emphysema; a variety of sounds include loud crackles, clicking, and gurgling sounds heard over the precordium; they are synchronous with the heartbeat and not particularly so with respirations.

18. _____: lower, more moist sound heard during the middle stage of inspiration and not cleared by a cough.

19. _____: dry, rubbing, or grating sound, usually caused by inflammation.

20. _____: low-pitched, low intensity sounds heard over healthy lung tissue.

Auscultation Sounds

1. On the illustration below, label the locations of the lung sounds you would expect to hear with auscultation of the anterior chest, using "B" for bronchial sounds, "BV" for bronchovesicular sounds, and "V" for vesicular sounds.
2. Mark the location of the manubrium with "M" and the angle of Louis with "AL."
3. Indicate the location of the costal angle with "CA."

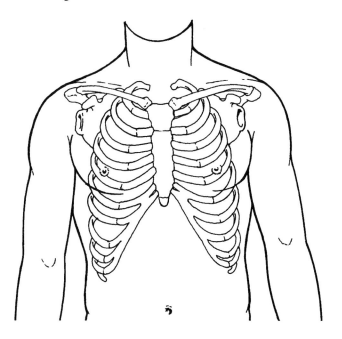

Examination Technique

For each clinical finding listed, identify the appropriate examination method that will elicit the finding.

Finding	Examination Method	Finding	Examination Method
Biot respiration		Bronchial	
Tactile fremitus		Rhonchi	
Cheyne-Stokes respiration		Barrel chest	
Dullness		Hyperresonance	
Vesicular		Wheezes	

Finding	Examination Method	Finding	Examination Method
Tympany		Tracheal tug	
Dyspnea		Crackles	
Bronchophony		Diaphragmatic excursion	
Vibration		Bronchovesicular	
Kussmaul breathing		Crepitus	

Matching

Match each examination finding with its corresponding diagnosis.

Examination Finding	Diagnosis
_____ 1. Airway reactivity triggered by allergens, anxiety, or upper respiratory infection	a. Bronchiectasis
_____ 2. Excessive nonpurulent fluid in the pleural space	b. Empyema
_____ 3. Inflammation of the mucous membranes of the bronchial tubes	c. Pulmonary embolism
_____ 4. Inflammatory process involving the visceral and parietal pleura	d. Asthma
_____ 5. Purulent exudate collected in the pleural spaces	e. Cystic fibrosis
_____ 6. Infection of the pulmonary parenchyma	f. Tuberculosis
_____ 7. Chronic infectious disease beginning in the lung with the tubercle bacillus	g. Pleurisy
_____ 8. Embolic occlusion of the pulmonary arteries	h. Bronchitis
_____ 9. Autosomal recessive disorder of the exocrine glands in children younger than 5 years of age	i. Pneumonia
_____ 10. Chronic dilation of the bronchi or bronchioles caused by repeated pulmonary infections	j. Pleural effusion

A 66-year-old woman presents with symptoms of shortness of breath. Listed below are initial data collected during an interview and examination.

INTERVIEW DATA

The patient states that she has had breathing problems "for years," but now they are getting worse. She tells the examiner that she gets short of breath with activity, adding that she can do things around the house for only a few minutes before she has to sit down to rest and catch her breath. She says that she can sleep only a couple of hours at a time. She sleeps best with two pillows at night but, on some nights, she just sits in a chair. She does not currently use oxygen, but she thinks oxygen would help. She admits to smoking 1½ packs of cigarettes a day. She has never quit because she says she just can't do it.

EXAMINATION DATA

General survey: Alert and slightly anxious woman, sitting slightly forward, with moderately labored breathing. Skin is pale, with slight cyanosis around the lips and in nail beds. Appears extremely thin.

Chest wall configuration: Chest is round shaped and symmetric, with an increased anteroposterior diameter and costal angle greater than 90 degrees. Small muscle mass noted over chest; ribs protrude.

Breathing effort: Respiratory rate 24 breaths/min and labored.

Chest assessment: Chest wall expansion with respirations is reduced but symmetric. Chest wall tactile fremitus diminished. Rhonchi are auscultated throughout lung field. Lung sounds are diminished in lung bases bilaterally.

Vocal sound auscultation: Muffled tones auscultated.

1. What data deviate from normal findings, suggesting a need for further investigation?

2. What additional questions could be asked by the examiner to clarify symptoms?

3. What additional physical examination, if any, should the examiner complete?

4. What type of problems do you anticipate that this patient will have?

1. A 72-year-old man is seen in the clinic for a routine examination. During the interview, he tells the interviewer that he smokes. When questioned further, he indicates that he has been smoking for "roughly 60 years." He states, "I started smoking cigarettes when I was about 14 years old. Until I was about 25, I smoked a pack maybe every 3 days or so. Then I started smoking about half a pack a day until the age of 40. Since that time, I've smoked almost a pack a day." He adds, "I knew I should quit, but I never really wanted to very much. I decided that when I got up to a pack a day, I would never smoke more than that." Based on the information given, calculate the patient's pack-year history.

2. A 41-year-old migrant worker from Mexico comes to the clinic where you work. Through an interpreter, you learn that he has had a fever with night sweats, fatigue, frequent coughing with reddish sputum, and weight loss. What significance do these symptoms have?

3. A mother of three tells you that all of her children have had problems with coughing and some trouble breathing ever since they moved into a new apartment 2 months ago. She says that they have not had fevers with these symptoms. What type of interview questions should be asked to further explore these symptoms?

Patient Safety Consideration

Which four symptoms indicate the need for immediate intervention because of severe upper airway obstruction?

CONTENT REVIEW QUESTIONS

Multiple Choice

Circle the best answer for each of the following questions:

1. As the chest of a newborn is examined, bowel sounds are auscultated in the chest. Which of the following best describes the significance of this finding?
   a. A normal finding in newborns
   b. An abnormal but benign finding in children until 2 years of age
   c. Abnormal and possibly indicating an enlarged liver
   d. Abnormal and possibly indicating a diaphragmatic hernia

2. Which of the following patients demonstrates the highest risk factor for respiratory disability?
   a. A patient with a history of hypertension
   b. A child who has had a previous respiratory infection
   c. A patient with paraplegia
   d. An extremely thin female patient

3. A healthcare professional is examining the chest of a 22-year-old woman who is 8 months pregnant. The patient has a wide thoracic cage. Which of the following best explains this finding?
   a. She may have lung disease, such as emphysema.
   b. She may be hypoxic and require oxygen supplementation.
   c. She may be pregnant with twins, causing abdominal contents to be forced up and out.
   d. This is considered a normal finding with advanced pregnancy.

4. In which of the following conditions should the examiner expect the costal angle to be greater than 90 degrees?
   a. Chronic obstructive pulmonary disease
   b. Pneumothorax
   c. Infant respiratory distress syndrome
   d. Atelectasis

77

5. Which of the following findings indicates respiratory distress in an infant or toddler?
   a. Respiratory rate of 30 breaths/min
   b. Hyperresonance of the chest
   c. Observation of sternal retractions with breathing
   d. Auscultation of bronchovesicular sounds throughout the lung field

6. During percussion, the patient is asked to "Fold your arms in front of you" in order to
   a. expose maximum lung area.
   b. make the ribs protrude.
   c. prevent attacks of coughing.
   d. reduce discomfort.

7. Which of the following examination techniques is *not* typically done when examining the chest and lungs of a newborn?
   a. Palpation
   b. Inspection
   c. Percussion
   d. Auscultation

8. The patient tells the examiner, "I have been coughing up a lot of yellowish-green phlegm." The examiner should suspect
   a. viral infection.
   b. tuberculosis.
   c. pulmonary edema.
   d. bacterial pneumonia.

9. To best visualize subtle retractions on a patient, the examiner should
   a. place the patient in a supine position.
   b. stand directly behind the patient.
   c. ensure that the light source angles toward the patient.
   d. position the patient directly under a bright examination light.

10. Which of the following findings may indicate a pulmonary infection?
    a. Malodorous breath
    b. Protrusion of the clavicle
    c. Clubbing of the nail beds
    d. Kussmaul respirations

11. Which finding is considered unusual for a newborn?
    a. Sneezing
    b. Coughing
    c. Silent hiccupping
    d. Nose breathing

12. In an older adult, which finding can occur in the absence of disease as a result of age-related changes of the chest or lungs?
    a. Barrel chest
    b. Productive cough
    c. Increased vital capacity
    d. Pulmonary infiltrate

13. Which symptom reported by a young adult indicates the need for questioning about cocaine use?
    a. Breathlessness at rest
    b. Expectoration of blood tinged mucus
    c. Severechest pain
    d. Inability to take deep breath

14. Hamman sign can best be heard when the patient is
    a. in a supine position.
    b. lying on the left side.
    c. sitting completely upright.
    d. positioned with the head elevated 30 degrees.

15. In addition to severe respiratory distress, which of the following findings may be indicative of a pneumothorax with mediastinal shift?
    a. Hemoptysis
    b. Pleural friction fremitus
    c. Vesicular lung sounds over the peripheral lung field
    d. Tracheal deviation away from midline position

16. A mother tells the examiner that her 2-year-old child has a cough that "sounds just like a bark." Given this history, what other findings should the examiner anticipate during respiratory examination?
    a. Wheezing and coarse crackles bilaterally
    b. Labored breathing and inspiratory stridor
    c. Hyperresonance with percussion
    d. Productive, blood-tinged, or "rusty" sputum

17. The examiner should expect the ratio of respiratory rate to heart rate in the adult to be approximately:
    a. 1 to 2.
    b. 1 to 4.
    c. 1 to 6.
    d. 1 to 8.

18. Which examination finding is consistent withpneumothorax?
    a. Decreased tactile fremitus
    b. Dullness with chest percussion
    c. Prolonged inspiration
    d. An ammonia-like odor to the patient's breath

19. The most important clinical signs for pleural effusion include which of the following?
    a. Bronchophony, yellow, frothy sputum
    b. Paroxysmal dyspnea, decreased breath sounds
    c. Shallow, rapid respirations
    d. Dullness to percussion, decreased tactile fremitus

20. Sounds associated with mediastinal emphysema are synchronous with
    a. heartbeat
    b. inspiration
    c. expiration
    d. swallowing

15 Heart

LEARNING OBJECTIVES

After studying Chapter 15 in the textbook and completing this section of the laboratory manual, students should be able to:

1. Describe anatomy and physiology of the heart.
2. Identify age and condition variations related to the heart.
3. Describe interview questions pertinent to the heart examination.
4. Discuss inspection, palpation, percussion, and auscultation techniques used for examination of the heart.
5. Describe age- and condition-specific variations in examination findings of the heart.
6. Identify examination findings associated with various conditions of the heart.

TERMINOLOGY REVIEW

Check your understanding of terminology related to assessment of the heart. Using the space provided, write the word or phrase from the list next to the appropriate descriptor.

Atria	Purkinje fibers
Diastole	Regurgitation
Heave	Septum
Intrinsic	Sinoatrial node
Myocardium	Still murmur
Pericardium	Systole
Point of maximal impulse (PMI)	Thrill
Pulmonic valve	

1. _____: a small mass of cardiac muscle fibers where the heart's impulse of stimulation originates.

2. _____: the location where the apical pulse is most readily seen or felt.

3. _____: referring to the type of electrical conduction system that enables the heart to contract and coordinates the sequence of muscular contractions taking place during the cardiac cycle.

4. _____: a fine, palpable sensation.

5. _____: fibers of the ventricular myocardium that are specialized cells for electrical conduction that conduct the electrical impulses in the heart.

6. _____: the phase of the cardiac cycle during which the ventricles dilate, drawing blood into the ventricles as the atria contract and thereby moving blood from the atria to the ventricles.

7. _____: small, thin-walled structures acting primarily as reservoirs for blood returning to the heart from the veins throughout the body.

8. _____: apical impulse that is more vigorous than expected.

9. _____: backward flow of blood.

10. _____: tough double-walled, fibrous sac encasing and protecting the heart.

11. _____: an auscultatory sound occurring in healthy children 3 to 7 years of age; caused by the vigorous expulsion of blood from the left ventricle into the aorta.

12. _____: structure that separates the right ventricle from the pulmonary artery.

13. _____: middle layer of the heart; responsible for the pumping action of the heart.

14. _____: partition dividing the left and right heart chambers.

15. _____: the contraction phase of the cardiac cycle.

APPLICATION TO CLINICAL PRACTICE

Anatomy Review

Identify the structures of the heart labeled on the illustration below. Using the list of terms provided, write the correct term in the blank next to the corresponding letter on the next page. Use each term once.

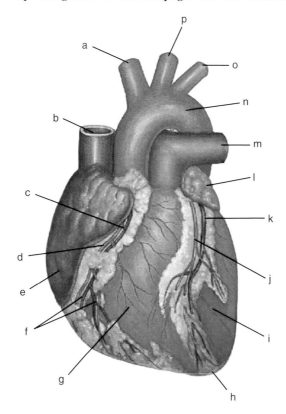

a. _____   Anterior cardiac veins

b. _____   Apex

c. _____   Arch of aorta

d. _____   Brachiocephalic artery

e. _____   Coronary sulcus

f. _____   Great cardiac vein

g. _____   Left atrium

h. _____   Left common carotid artery

i. _____   Left coronary artery

j. _____   Left pulmonary artery

k. _____   Left subclavian artery

l. _____   Left ventricle

m. _____   Right atrium

n. _____   Right coronary artery

o. _____   Right ventricle

p. _____   Superior vena cava

CONCEPTS APPLICATION

Complete the following table by indicating where you would auscultate to locate each valve listed.

Valve	Where Would You Auscultate?
Tricuspid valve	
Mitral valve	
Aortic valve	
Pulmonic valve	

Matching

Match each examination finding with its corresponding diagnosis.

Examination Finding	Diagnosis
_____ 1. Increase in mass and lateral displacement of the left ventricle	a. Ventricular septal defect
_____ 2. Bacterial infection of the endothelial layer of the heart	b. Angina
_____ 3. Syndrome in which the heart fails to propel blood forward	c. Congestive heart failure
_____ 4. Inflammation of the pericardium	d. Pericarditis
_____ 5. Sinoatrial node dysfunction	e. Sick sinus syndrome
_____ 6. Elevated serum cholesterol	f. Aortic stenosis
_____ 7. Opening between the left and right ventricles	g. Left ventricular hypertrophy
_____ 8. Systemic connective tissue disease that commonly occurs after streptococcal infection	h. Acute rheumatic fever
_____ 9. Substernal pain or intense pressure	i. Bacterial endocarditis
_____ 10. Thickening and calcification of the aortic valve	j. Hyperlipidemia

Case Study

A 76-year-old man comes to the clinic because of difficulty in breathing. Listed below are initial data collected during an interview and examination.

INTERVIEW DATA

The patient doesn't know exactly when his breathing difficulty started, but it has gotten noticeably worse the past couple of days. He volunteers at the church library three mornings a week and plays golf twice a week. However, he says that this past week, he has "just felt too tired to do anything." He also says that he has not been able to sleep very well at night because of his breathing difficulty. He adds, "I keep coughing out this frothy-looking phlegm." He denies taking any medications at this time. He says that he doesn't smoke or drink alcoholic beverages.

EXAMINATION DATA

General survey: Alert, cooperative, well-groomed man. Appears to be stated age. Breathing is mildly labored.

Vital signs: Temperature 98.8°F (37.1°C); pulse 120 beats/min; respirations 26 breaths/min; BP 142/112 right arm, 144/110 left arm.

Pulses: All pulses palpable 2+ . No carotid bruits bilaterally.

Lower extremities: Skin warm and dry without cyanosis. Even hair distribution. 2+ pitting edema noted bilaterally. No lesions present.

Neck: Jugular distention and pulsation noted with patient in supine position.

1. What data deviate from normal findings, suggesting a need for further investigation?

2. What additional questions could be asked by the examiner to clarify symptoms?

3. What additional physical examination, if any, should the examiner complete?

4. What type of problems do you anticipate that this patient will have?

CLINICAL REASONING

1. A mother tells you that her 2½-year-old son prefers to squat while watching TV rather than to sit on the couch or floor. What is the potential significance of this statement?

2. A 10-year-old girl is brought to the clinic by her mother. The mother tells the examiner that the girl has been very tired and short of breath and that she has been running a low-grade fever. These symptoms have been getting progressively worse over the past few weeks. The only significant health history is treatment for strep throat last month. What, specifically, should the examiner look for to aid in the diagnosis?

3. A 42-year-old Native American or American Indian man with insulin-dependent diabetes mellitus (IDDM is seen in the clinic for a diabetic foot ulcer that does not heal. In what ways does IDDM increase his risk for cardiovascular-related problems?

Patient Safety Consideration
In older adults, the cardiac response to even minimal demand may be slowed or insufficient. As a result, transient light-headedness may occur with position change because of a drop in arterial pressure. What precautions can you take during your physical examination of an older adult to protect against injury related to this type of event?

Multiple Choice

Circle the best answer for each of the following questions:

1. Dextrocardia is a condition characterized by which of the following?
   a. The right side of the heart is enlarged.
   b. The heart is positioned to the right of the stomach.
   c. The heart is positioned to the right, either rotated or displaced.
   d. Blood glucose level in the heart is higher than in other organs.

2. While auscultating the heart of an obese patient, the examiner should expect the heart sounds to be
   a. louder and closer.
   b. softer and more distant.
   c. louder and more distant.
   d. softer and closer.

3. What disease process should the examiner consider if a patient reports a history of fever and has sudden onset of clinical symptoms of congestive heart failure?
   a. Bacterial endocarditis
   b. Infarction
   c. Myocarditis
   d. Cardiac tamponade

4. The examiner suspects that a patient has pulmonary hypertension. What examination findings are consistent with this?
   a. Decreased intensity of S1 heart sounds; increased intensity of S2 heart sounds
   b. A thrill palpated in the area of apex
   c. Paradoxic splitting of S1 and S2 heart sounds
   d. Pericardial friction rub

5. Which of the following cardiac changes occurs at birth in the normal child?
   a. The foramen ovale opens.
   b. Pressure in the right atrium rises.
   c. The ductus arteriosus closes.
   d. The relative mass of the left ventricle decreases.

6. In most adults, the apical impulse should be visible at the
   a. midaxillary line in the fifth right intercostal space.
   b. sternal notch.
   c. midclavicular line in the fifth left intercostal space.
   d. costovertebral angle.

7. While palpating the precordium, a heave is identified, with lateral displacement of the apical pulse. Such a finding may indicate
   a. mitral regurgitation.
   b. aortic stenosis.
   c. left ventricular hypertrophy.
   d. pericarditis.

8. A thrill generally indicates which of the following?
   a. A disturbance in the electrical conductivity of the heart
   b. A fine, rushing vibration related to disruption of blood flow in the heart
   c. The presence of significant infection of the myocardium
   d. Forceful apical impulse felt below the left sternal border

9. Because percussion has a limited value in determining heart size, left ventricular size is more accurately determined by
   a. auscultating the heart sounds.
   b. locating the apical pulse or PMI.
   c. palpating the left sternal border.
   d. palpating the heart base.

10. Which of the following may be easily mistaken for cardiac-generated sounds?
    a. Bowel sounds
    b. Pulmonary insufficiency
    c. Pericardial friction rub
    d. Tracheal shifting

11. Cardiac tamponade is
    a. caused by myocardial infarct and requires immediate intervention.
    b. indicated by jugular venous distention, hypertension, and exaggerated heart sounds.
    c. the result of excessive accumulation of fluid between the pericardium and the heart.
    d. characterized by excessive cardiac relaxation, increased blood pressure, and bounding pulse.

12. During cardiac auscultation, the examiner notes a midsystolic murmur with a medium pitch; a coarse thrill is palpated as well. These findings are consistent with which condition?
    a. Aortic stenosis
    b. Aortic regurgitation
    c. Pulmonic stenosis
    d. Mitral stenosis

13. Which physical finding is most suggestive of right-sided heart failure?
    a. Cardiomegaly
    b. Hypotension
    c. Jugular venous distention
    d. Shortness of breath

14. Which of the following cardiovascular findings would be considered normal for a woman who is 8 months pregnant?
    a. The apical impulse has shifted upward and laterally.
    b. Splitting of S1 and S2 is less audible.
    c. A grade III diastolic ejection murmur is heard.
    d. A fourth heart sound can be auscultated.

15. Which principle helps the examiner determine where heart sounds are best heard?
    a. The Doppler effect diminishes the sound over time.
    b. Sound is transmitted in the direction of blood flow.
    c. Accumulation of fluid magnifies the intensity of sound.
    d. Duration of sound varies directly with frequency.

16. S_2 is
    a. the result of opening of the atrioventricular valves.
    b. the beginning of systole.
    c. best heard in the mitral area.
    d. of higher pitch and shorter duration than S_1.

17. Splitting of heart sounds is
    a. an unexpected event that should be further evaluated.
    b. the result of opening of the valves during inspiration.
    c. Often most distinct at the end of expiration.
    d. caused by desynchronized valve closure.

18. To distinguish a heart murmur from respiratory sounds in an infant, the examiner could correctly do which of the following?
    a. Time the sound with the carotid pulsation.
    b. Distract the child with a moving toy.
    c. Ask the child to hold his or her breath.
    d. Use the flat side of the stethoscope to auscultate the child's chest.

19. In a young child, the examiner notes a systolic ejection murmur that is loud, harsh, and high in pitch heard over the second intercostal space along the left sternal border. What problem should the examiner suspect?
    a. Mitral valve prolapse
    b. Mitral valve stenosis
    c. Coarctation of the aorta
    d. Atrial septal defect

20. To hear low-pitched filling sounds of the heart, the examiner should place the patient in a
    a. supine position and listen with the bell of the stethoscope.
    b. sitting position and listen with the diaphragm of the stethoscope.
    c. sitting position and listen with the bell of the stethoscope.
    d. left lateral recumbent position and listen with the bell of the stethoscope.

16 Blood Vessels

LEARNING OBJECTIVES

After studying Chapter 16 in the textbook and completing this section of the laboratory manual, students should be able to:

1. Describe anatomy and physiology of the blood vessels.
2. Identify age and condition variations in the blood vessels.
3. Describe interview questions pertinent to an examination of the blood vessels.
4. Discuss inspection, palpation, percussion, and auscultation techniques for examination of the blood vessels.
5. Describe age- and condition-specific variations in examination findings of the blood vessels.
6. Identify examination findings associated with various conditions of the blood vessels.

TERMINOLOGY REVIEW

Check your understanding of terminology related to the blood vessels. Using the space provided, write the word or phrase from the list next to the appropriate descriptor.

Arterial aneurysm	**Pitting**
Arterial embolic disease	**Raynaud phenomenon**
Arteriovenous fistula	**Regurgitation**
Bruit	**Varicose veins**
Claudication	**Venous thrombosis**
Hum	**Venous ulcers**
Jugular Pulse Wave	
Peripheral arterial disease	

1. _____: dilated and swollen veins with a diminished rate of blood flow and increased intravenous pressure; result from the incompetence of the vessel wall or venous valves or an obstruction in the more proximal vein.

2. _____: a venous phenomenon without pathologic significance that is common in children.

3. _____: decreased on inspiration and increased on expiration and more prominent with increased abdominal pressure.

4. _____: pain resulting from muscle ischemia, characterized by a dull ache with accompanying muscle fatigue and cramps.

5. _____: a blood clot that forms within a vein, which can occur suddenly or gradually and with varying severity of symptoms; can be the result of trauma or prolonged immobilization.

6. _____: a condition in which emboli are dispersed throughout the arterial system; emboli can be caused by a thrombus, atherosclerotic plaques, infectious material from fungal and bacterial endocarditis, or atrial myxomas (a mass of connective tissue).

7. _____: exaggerated spasms of the digital arterioles (occasionally in the nose and ears), usually in response to cold exposure.

8. _____: result from chronic venous insufficiency in which lack of venous flow leads to lower extremity venous hypertension.

9. _____: murmur or unexpected sound, usually low pitched and relatively hard to hear.

10. _____: a type of edema characterized by a dent or depression that does not rapidly refill and resume its original contour.

11. _____: a pathologic communication between an artery and a vein; may be congenital or acquired.

12. _____: a localized dilation, generally defined as 1.5 times the diameter of the normal artery, caused by the weakness in the arterial wall.

13. _____: stenosis of the blood vessels supplying blood to the extremities; most often caused by atherosclerotic plaques but can also be a result of vascular trauma, radiation therapy, or vasculitis.

14. _____: backflow of blood as a result of incompetent valves.

APPLICATION TO CLINICAL PRACTICE

Anatomy Review

Identify the arterial pulse sites labeled on the diagram by writing the correct term in the blank.

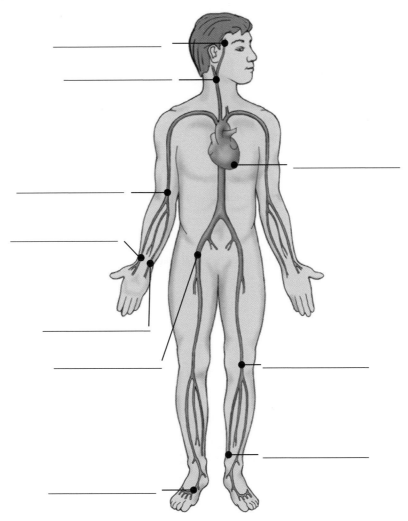

From Bonewit-West K, Hunt SA, Applegate E. *Today's Medical Assistant: Clinical & Administrative Procedures*, 3rd ed. St. Louis, MO: Elsevier, 2016.

Concepts Application Activity 1

Based on the location of pain, identify the probable obstructed artery.

Location of Pain	Probable Obstructed Artery
Calf muscles	
Thigh	
Buttock	

Concepts Application Activity 2

Complete the columns below by describing three characteristics that differentiate the pain of arterial insufficiency from the pain of venous insufficiency or musculoskeletal disorders.

Arterial Insufficiency	Venous Insufficiency or Musculoskeletal Disorders
1.	
2.	
3.	

Matching

Match each examination finding with its corresponding diagnosis.

Examination Finding	Diagnosis
_____ 1. Generalized inflammatory disease of the branches of the aortic arch	a. Preeclampsia
_____ 2. Idiopathic, intermittent spasm of the arterioles in the digits	b. Ulnar artery insufficiency
_____ 3. Abnormal Allen test	c. Venous thrombosis
_____ 4. Tenderness along the iliac vessels and femoral canal	d. Temporal arteritis
_____ 5. Holosystolic murmur in the region of tricuspid valve	e. Raynaud phenomenon
_____ 6. Congenital stenosis in the descending aortic arch in children	f. Venous ulcers
_____ 7. Hypertension that occurs after the 20th week of pregnancy along with the presence of proteinuria	g. Coarctation of the aorta
_____ 8. Chronic venous insufficiency in which lack of venous flow leads to lower extremity venous hypertension	h. Tricuspid regurgitation

Case Study

A 32-year-old woman presents with symptoms of pain in her fingers, with more discomfort in her dominant right hand. Listed below are initial data collected during an interview and examination.

<u>INTERVIEW DATA</u>

The patient began to notice changes in her hands about 3 months ago when she started a new job where she spends several hours a day at a computer keyboard. Since then, the pain has steadily increased, and she is alarmed about the development of a dark spot on the tip of the fifth finger of her right hand. She attends aerobic classes weekly but is not able to keep up with the class because of shortness of breath. She has smoked a pack of cigarettes daily for the past 10 years. She has a moderate alcohol intake of two to three glasses of wine per week. She is taking no medications at this time.

<u>EXAMINATION DATA</u>

General survey: Alert, cooperative, well-groomed woman who appears to be her stated age. Shortness of breath noted upon reaching the examination room but abated after 1 minute of rest.

Vital signs: Temperature 98.8°F (37.1°C). Pulse 100 beats/min on arrival to room; 76 beats/min after 5 minutes. BP 126/82 in both arms.

Pulses: All pulses palpable, 2+. Fingers on both hands cool to touch.

Lower extremities: Skin warm and dry; free of cyanosis or erythema. Hair distribution is even. No edema noted. No lesions present.

Upper extremities: Fingers cool, capillary refill sluggish. Dark lesion noted on tip of right fifth finger, 4 mm in diameter. Some reduced range of motion noted in both hands. Skin over the hands appears tight and probably contributes to the reduced range of motion.

Neck: Supple. No neck vein distention noted.

1. What data deviate from normal findings, suggesting a need for further investigation?

2. What additional questions could the examiner ask to clarify symptoms?

3. What additional physical examination, if any, should the examiner complete?

4. What type of problems do you anticipate this patient will have?

1. A patient reports that he has increasing pain in the calf of his left leg, which he began to notice after a long airplane ride 1 month ago. He is 56 years old and has smoked a half a pack of cigarettes a day for the past 20 years. Examination reveals some redness and tenderness over the affected area. What do these symptoms suggest, and what is the patient at risk for?

2. A woman comes to her routine prenatal check at 32 weeks' gestation complaining of difficulty with dizziness when she gets up from bed or from a seated position. What is the most likely cause of her symptoms?

Patient Safety Consideration

What must the examiner NEVER do when examining the carotid arteries? Why?

CONTENT REVIEW QUESTIONS

Multiple Choice

Circle the best answer for each of the following questions:

1. The carotid artery is considered the most suitable artery for evaluation of cardiac function because it
   a. is the largest artery in the peripheral vascular system.
   b. is the most pliable artery in the peripheral vascular system.
   c. is the most accessible artery close to the heart.
   d. has the thickest layer of smooth muscle within the vessel walls.

2. The purpose of the great vessels is to
   a. provide a reservoir for blood volume to be used in times of stress.
   b. circulate the blood to and from the body and the lungs.
   c. quickly and efficiently move blood in and out of the heart.
   d. send blood to the lungs for large-scale reoxygenation.

3. Pregnant women may experience palmar erythema and spider telangiectasis as a result of
   a. peripheral vasodilation with decreased vascular resistance.
   b. peripheral vasoconstriction.
   c. increased peripheral resistance.
   d. diminished cardiac output and peripheral vascular resistance.

4. Why would an examiner perform an Allen test on a patient?
   a. To evaluate risk of thrombophlebitis
   b. To detect cyclic differences in the pulse wave
   c. To check patency of the ulnar artery
   d. To monitor for development of a bruit

5. A bounding pulse would be expected in an infant with what condition?
   a. Coarctation of the aorta
   b. Patent ductus arteriosus
   c. Venous hum
   d. Right-sided heart failure

6. Which word best describes a 3+ amplitude pulse?
   a. Diminished
   b. Normal
   c. Full
   d. Bounding

7. Claudication
   a. indicates tissue necrosis caused by venous insufficiency.
   b. is pain that results from muscle ischemia.
   c. progresses from a sharp, tingling pain to a dull, burning ache.
   d. occurs after exercise and during sleep.

8. Which action will diminish the intensity of a venous hum?
   a. Tilting the head slightly upward
   b. Turning the head away from the area of auscultation
   c. Performing the Valsalva maneuver
   d. Taking a deep breath

9. Which characteristic of the pulse is being described when the pulse is referred to as bounding?
   a. Regularity
   b. Amplitude
   c. Contour
   d. Waveform

10. How does rotating the patient's head to the side being examined facilitate palpation of the carotid pulse?
    a. It "fixes" the artery in place.
    b. It increases the pulse amplitude.
    c. It brings the artery closer to the skin surface.
    d. It relaxes the sternocleidomastoid muscle.

11. Hepatojugular reflux can be used to evaluate
    a. right-sided heart failure.
    b. degree of aortic stenosis.
    c. incompetence of venous valves.
    d. arterial insufficiency.

12. In determining the jugular venous pressure, the examiner would correctly do which of the following?
    a. Apply manual pressure on the carotid artery while the patient forcefully exhales.
    b. Examine neck veins while occluding the brachial artery with the blood pressure cuff.
    c. Use light to supply tangential illumination across the neck.
    d. Have the patient lean forward from the waist and take a deep breath.

13. Varicose veins are characterized by
    a. dilation and tortuosity when the extremities are dependent.
    b. increased rate of blood flow to the extremities.
    c. decreased intravenous pressure.
    d. edema resulting from obstruction to a distal vein.

14. A condition that results in progressive ischemia caused by insufficient perfusion is
    a. Raynaud phenomenon.
    b. peripheral atherosclerotic disease.
    c. venous thrombosis.
    d. arterial aneurysm.

15. Which problem should be suspected when an examiner documents that a patient has " thickened skin and 2+ pitting edema of the right lower extremity"?
    a. Lymphedema
    b. Arterial insufficiency
    c. Occlusion of a major vein
    d. Congestive heart failure

16. Which is a characteristic of the jugular pulse that can aid the examiner in differentiating it from the carotid pulse?
    a. The jugular pulse can be visualized but not palpated.
    b. Respiration has no effect on the jugular pulse.
    c. Pressure on the left upper quadrant of the abdomen will obliterate the jugular pulse.
    d. Exaggeration of the jugular pulse occurs in response to pressure just above the clavicle.

17. The most common cause of venous thrombosis in children is
    a. congenital venous incompetence.
    b. atherosclerosis of deep veins.
    c. arteriovenous malformation.
    d. placement of venous access devices.

18. Which fact is critical for an examiner to consider when evaluating a patient with a possible deep vein thrombosis (DVT)?
    a. A defining characteristic of DVT is venous distention after five deep knee bends.
    b. DVT cannot be confirmed based solely on physical examination.
    c. A negative Homan sign rules out the diagnosis of DVT.
    d. It is impossible to distinguish Achilles tendon pain from DVT on clinical examination.

19. Which of the following distinguishes musculoskeletal pain from the pain of vascular insufficiency?
    a. Onset during activity
    b. Increases with intensity and duration of activity
    c. May occur several hours after activity
    d. Quickly relieved by rest

20. When examining a 10-month-old infant, the examiner should suspect dehydration or hypovolemic shock when capillary refill time is longer than ___ second(s).
    a. 1
    b. 2
    c. 3
    d. 4

LEARNING OBJECTIVES

After studying Chapter 17 in the textbook and completing this section of the laboratory manual, students should be able to:
1. Conduct a history related to the breasts and axillae.
2. Discuss examination techniques for the breasts and axillae.
3. Identify normal age- and condition-related variations of the breasts and axillae.
4. Recognize findings that deviate from expected findings.
5. Relate symptoms or clinical findings to common pathologic conditions.

TERMINOLOGY REVIEW

Check your understanding of terminology related to the breasts and axillae. Using the space provided, write the word or phrase from the list next to the appropriate descriptor.

Areola	Mammogram
Colostrum	Montgomery follicles
Cooper ligaments	Peau d'orange appearance
Duct ectasia	Thelarche
Fat necrosis	Tail of Spence
Galactorrhea	Tanner staging
Gynecomastia	Virchow nodes
Involution	

1. _____: breast enlargement, first sign of puberty in females.

2. _____: suspensory structures which along with the layer of sub-cutaneous fibrous tissue provide support for the breast.

3. _____: tiny, raised sebaceous glands which commonly appear in the areola; also called tubercles.

4. _____: lymph nodes considered to be sentinel nodes for signaling lymphatic invasion of carcinoma.

5. _____: benign breast lump that occurs as an inflammatory response to local injury; necrotic fat and cellular debris become fibrotic and may contract into a scar.

6. _____: breast tissue which extends from the upper outer quadrant of the breast into the axilla.

7. _____: pigmented area surrounding the nipple that should be round or oval and bilaterally symmetric or nearly so; the color ranges from pink to black.

8. _____: enlargement of breast tissue in men.

9. _____: a common radiologic procedure used for breast examination.

10. _____: method to determine level of sexual maturity which can be used to stage breast development.

11. _____: lactation not associated with childbearing, usually from elevated levels of prolactin, resulting in milk production.

12. _____: benign condition of the subareolar ducts that produces nipple discharge; the subareolar ducts become dilated and blocked with desquamating secretory epithelium necrotic debris and chronic inflammatory cells.

13. _____: clear or milky-white fluid expressed from the breast before milk production; it contains antibodies and also more protein and minerals than mature milk does.

14. _____: the interval, usually about 3 months, after termination of lactation when the breasts decrease in size.

15. _____: appearance of this indicates edema of the breast caused by blocking lymph drainage in advance of inflammatory breast cancer; the skin appears thickened, with enlarged pores and accentuated skin markings.

APPLICATION TO CLINICAL PRACTICE

Matching
Match each clinical finding with its corresponding associated factor or cause.

Clinical Finding	Associated Factor or Cause
_____ 1. Galactorrhea	a. Thickened inframammary ridge
_____ 2. Mastitis	b. Usually worse premenstrually
_____ 3. Fibrocystic disease	c. Often regresses after menopause
_____ 4. Expected postmenopausal change	d. Administration of phenothiazines
_____ 5. Fibroadenoma	e. Often associated with a clogged milk duct
_____ 6. Orange skin	f. Blocked subareolar ducts
_____ 7. Paget disease	g. Red, scaling, crusty patch on nipple
_____ 8. Mammary duct ectasia	h. Blocked lymph drainage

Concepts Application
On the illustrations below, draw the direction of palpation that the examiner would use for the (a) concentric circles technique, (b) wedge technique, and (c) vertical striptechnique.

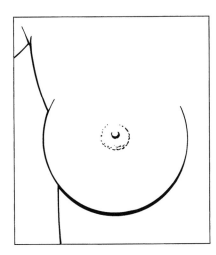 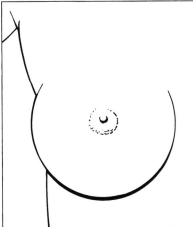 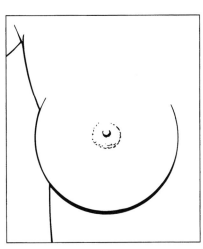

A 46-year-old woman comes to the clinic because she has discovered a lump in her left breast. Listed below are data collected during an interview and examination.

INTERVIEW DATA

The patient tells the examiner that she first noticed the lump about 9 months ago. Because the lump seemed small and did not hurt, she did not think it was much to worry about. Recently, she noted that the lump felt bigger and decided she better have someone look at it. She tells the examiner, "I just know it is not cancer because I am much too young and healthy. And if it is, I am not about to let some doctor mutilate me with a knife. I'd rather die than have my breast cut off." The examiner asks her whether she has noticed any redness or dimpling of the breast. She replies, "No, not really, but I don't pay attention to those sorts of things." She tells the examiner that she started having regular menstrual cycles at the age of 11 years and has not reached menopause. She has never been married and has no children.

EXAMINATION DATA

General survey: Very nervous, well-nourished woman. Is hesitant to expose her breast for examination.

Breast examination: Inspection reveals breasts of typical size with right and left breast symmetry. The skin of both breasts is smooth, with even pigmentation. The nipples protrude slightly with no drainage noted. The left nipple is slightly retracted. Significant dimpling is noted on the left breast in the upper outer quadrant when the arms are raised over her head. The right breast appears normal. Palpation of the left breast reveals a large, hard lump in the upper outer quadrant. No lumps or masses are noted in the right breast. The left nipple produces a clear, bloody-type discharge when squeezed; the right nipple is unremarkable.

1. What data deviate from normal findings, suggesting a need for further investigation?

2. What additional questions could the examiner ask to clarify symptoms?

3. What additional physical examination, if any, should the examiner complete?

4. What primary problems does the patient have?

CLINICAL REASONING

1. A 43-year-old female patient tells you that her mother died of breast cancer and her 50-year-old sister currently has breast cancer. She is worried about developing breast cancer as well. Her gynecologic history includes menarche at age 11 years. She has one child, a 7-year-old son. She has no history of other pregnancies and no history of illness. List her current risk factors. Would you consider her to be at increased risk for breast cancer? Explain your rationale.

2. A 50-year-old woman asks if you can help her "understand what is going on with breast screening guidelines." She says, "It seems like everything I was taught all my life has changed." What information would you use in formulating your response?

CONTENT REVIEW QUESTIONS

Multiple Choice

Circle the best answer for each of the following questions.

1. Which characteristic suggests that a lesion on a patient's breast is Paget disease and *not* eczema?
   a. Itchy predominantly at night
   b. Erythematous and crusty
   c. Confined to the nipple and areola of one breast
   d. Does not respond to steroids

2. How should a breast examination on a patient who had a lumpectomy for breast cancer *differ* from a breast examination on a patient who has not had breast cancer?
   a. Supraclavicular and infraclavicular lymph nodes are palpated.
   b. The lateral position with hands over the head is used for palpation.
   c. The area of the scar is palpated with two fingers using a circular motion.
   d. The fingertips are used to palpate for intercostal breast tissue.

3. While palpating the axilla, it is best to place the patient in a
   a. sitting position with the arm flexed at the elbow.
   b. sitting position with the arm at the side.
   c. supine position with the arms on the hips.
   d. lateral position with the arms at the sides.

4. Nipple compression should be included as part of the breast examination for which of the following patients?
   a. A 23-year-old woman concerned about "lumps and tenderness" premenstrually
   b. A 35-year-old lactating woman with "very sore nipples"
   c. A 48-year-old woman reporting two episodes of bloody discharge from the right nipple
   d. A 60-year-old man with gynecomastia

5. A supernumerary nipple is found on a white newborn infant girl. Which of the following may accompany this finding?
   a. Increased risk for breast cancer as an adult
   b. Increased lactation volume as an adult
   c. Congenital renal or cardiac anomalies
   d. Mental retardation

6. Which are typical descriptors of fibroadenoma?
   a. Bilateral, stellate, rubbery, nontender
   b. Multiple, unilateral, tender, well defined
   c. Single, discoid, firm, nontender
   d. Unilateral, hard, stellate, fixed

7. Which is the correct position in which to place a patient for breast palpation?
   a. Supine with the arms at the sides and a pillow under the neck
   b. Supine with the arm over the head and a small pillow under the shoulder of the side being assessed
   c. Left lateral position with the arm bent backward
   d. Sitting slightly forward with the breasts hanging away from the chest; the hands on the hips

8. Which statement made by a 37-year-old woman would make the examiner suspect fibrocystic disease?
   a. "I have a lump in my breast that is not tender."
   b. "My right breast is larger than my left breast."
   c. "My nipples are darker than before my baby was born."
   d. "I feel a lump in my breast before my period."

9. A patient, 3 weeks postpartum, tells the examiner that she is currently breastfeeding but might stop because her nipples are sore. The examiner observes dry and cracked nipples. Which of the following questions would be helpful in gaining information relevant to treating the problem?
   a. "Do you pump your breasts?"
   b. "How do you clean your breasts?"
   c. "Have you been able to bond with your infant?"
   d. "What medications have you been taking?"

10. A 68-year-old man presents with gynecomastia. Which factor is a potential cause of the problem?
    a. A decrease in physical activity
    b. Increased lactiferous duct glands
    c. Lymphatic engorgement
    d. A decrease in testosterone

11. Symptoms consistent with underlying ductal malignancy include
    a. erythema, heat, and pain over and around one nipple.
    b. red, scaling, crusty patch on one nipple.
    c. bilateral inflammation; tenderness; and sticky, multicolored nipple discharge.
    d. gynecomastia and a deepening color of the nipple.

12. While examining the breast of a 52-year-old woman, the examiner notes nipple discharge. Which of the following diagnostic tests would be appropriate?
    a. Cytologic examination of the discharge
    b. Culture and sensitivity examination of the discharge
    c. White blood cell count
    d. Estrogen level

13. While performing a breast examination on a 68-year-old woman, the examiner would expect which of the following findings?
    a. The breast tissue has multiple large, firm lumps in it.
    b. The breast tissue has a granular feel to it.
    c. The tail of Spence is no longer observed.
    d. The axillary lymph nodes are enlarged.

14. Which of the following represents the first sign of puberty in girls?
    a. Thelarche
    b. Menarche
    c. Proliferation of lactiferous duct
    d. Areolar elevation

15. A benign tumor of the subareolar duct that produces nipple discharge is
    a. Paget disease.
    b. intraductal papilloma.
    c. duct ectasia.
    d. galactorrhea.

16. A 38-year-old woman is diagnosed with mastitis. What is the likely causative agent?
    a. *Staphylococcus aureus*
    b. *Streptococcus aureus*
    c. *Neisseria gonorrhoeae*
    d. *Escherichia coli*

17. Which finding on examination of a female patient's breasts requires further investigation?
    a. Wrinkled areolas
    b. Prominent Montgomery tubercles
    c. One breast larger than the other
    d. Unilateral visible venous network

18. Which finding on breast examination of a male patient can result from marijuana use?
    a. Galactorrhea
    b. Subareolar mass
    c. Gynecomastia
    d. Dimpling

18 Abdomen

LEARNING OBJECTIVES

After studying Chapter 18 in the textbook and completing this section of the laboratory manual, students should be able to:
1. Conduct a history related to the abdomen.
2. Discuss examination techniques for the abdomen.
3. Identify normal age- and condition-related variations of the abdomen.
4. Recognize findings that deviate from expected findings.
5. Relate symptoms or clinical findings to common pathologic conditions.

TERMINOLOGY REVIEW

Check your understanding of terminology related to examination of the abdomen. Using the space provided, write the word or phrase from the list next to the appropriate descriptor.

Ascites
Ballottement
Borborygmi
Colic
Hydronephrosis
Intussusception
Mesentery
Pepsin
Peristalsis
Peritoneum

Pylorus
Reflux
Renal calculi
Scaphoid abdomen
Striae
Tympany
Volvulus

1. _____: spasmodic pains in the abdomen.

2. _____: commonly known as "stretch marks."

3. _____: a concave contour of the abdomen; a sign that suggests diaphragmatic hernia in the newborn.

4. _____: fan-shaped fold of peritoneum that anchors the small intestine to the abdominal wall.

5. _____: distal section of the stomach.

6. _____: muscular contractions that move the products of digestion through the alimentary canal.

7. _____: loud, prolonged gurgles.

8. _____: low-pitched, resonant, drumlike sound obtained by percussing the surface of a large, air-containing body space.

9. _____: backflow caused by relaxation or incompetence of the lower esophagus.

10. _____: Dilation of the renal pelvis and calyces due to an obstruction of urine flow anywhere from the urethral meatus to the kidneys

97

11. _____: twisting of the intestine, resulting in an obstruction.

12. _____: serous membrane lining the abdominal cavity.

13. _____: a palpation technique used to assess an organ or a mass.

14. _____: an enzyme that acts to digest proteins.

15. _____: a pathologic increase in fluid in the peritoneal cavity; may be suspected in the patient with risk factors.

16. _____: prolapse or telescoping of one segment of intestine into another, causing intestinal obstruction; commonly occurs in infants between 3 and 12 months of age.

17. _____: stones formed in the pelvis of the kidney as a result of a physiochemical process; associated with obstruction and infections in the urinary tract.

APPLICATION TO CLINICAL PRACTICE

Anatomy Review

Identify the structures of the abdomen labeled on the illustration below by writing the correct term in the blank next to the corresponding letter on the next page. Use each term once.

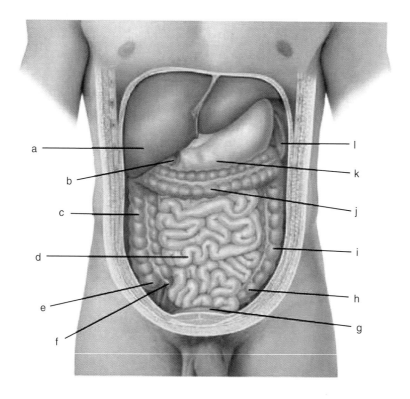

a. _____	Appendix
b. _____	Ascending colon
c. _____	Bladder
d. _____	Cecum
e. _____	Descending colon
f. _____	Gallbladder
g. _____	Liver
h. _____	Small intestine
i. _____	Sigmoid colon
j. _____	Spleen
k. _____	Stomach
l. _____	Transverse colon

Matching 1

Match each clinical finding with its corresponding abdominal condition.

Clinical Finding	Abdominal Condition
____ 1. Knifelike pain	a. Intraabdominal infectious process
____ 2. Dark-yellow urine	b. Ulcer
____ 3. Pain with gradual onset	c. Liver or biliary disease
____ 4. Colic pain	d. Pancreatitis
____ 5. Bruit	e. Renal stone
____ 6. Burning pain	f. Aortic aneurysm

Concepts Application 1

Consider the two recognized divisions of the abdomen: four quadrants of the abdomen and nine regions of the abdomen. Referring to the illustration in the Anatomy Review exercise, identify on the chart below the quadrant and the region where each of the listed abdominal structures are located. (Some structures are found in more than one quadrant or region.) The first one has been completed for you.

Structure	Quadrant	Region
Appendix	Right lower quadrant	Right inguinal
Colon		
Gallbladder		
Liver		
Pancreas		
Small intestine		
Spleen		
Stomach		

Concepts Application 2

Complete the table below to compare and contrast types of pain, abdominal signs, and associated symptoms or findings with the various conditions.

Condition	Type of Pain	Abdominal Signs	Associated Symptoms or Findings
Peritonitis	Sudden or gradual onset of generalized or localized pain described as dull to severe; increase in pain with deep inspirations		
		+Murphy sign	
Ectopic pregnancy			Symptoms of pregnancy, spotting, hypogastric tenderness, mass on bimanual pelvic examination; with rupture: shock, rigid abdominal wall distention
	Sudden and dramatic LUQ, umbilical, or epigastric pain that may be referred to left shoulder		Fever, epigastric tenderness, vomiting
		+Kehr sign	Fever, hematuria

Concepts Application 3

Several sounds are heard on auscultation. For each sound listed below, identify the possible associated condition.

Sound on Auscultation	Possible Associated Condition
Increased bowel sounds	
High-pitched tinkling sounds	
Decreased bowel sounds	
Friction rub	
Venous hum	

Matching 2

Match each clinical finding with its corresponding diagnosis.

Clinical Finding	Diagnosis
_____ 1. Relaxation or incompetence of the lower esophageal sphincter	a. Cirrhosis
_____ 2. Part of the stomach passing through the esophageal hiatus	b. Pyloric stenosis
_____ 3. Abdominal pain, bloating, constipation, and diarrhea	c. Irritable bowel syndrome
_____ 4. Ulceration, fibrosis, and malabsorption from an inflammatory disorder	d. Cholelithiasis
_____ 5. Left lower quadrant pain, anorexia, nausea, vomiting, possible constipation	e. Gastroesophageal reflux
	f. Renal abscess
_____ 6. Stone formation in the gallbladder	g. Diverticulitis
_____ 7. Destruction of the liver parenchyma	h. Hiatal hernia
_____ 8. Positive Blumberg, Markle and Balance signs along with obturator and iliopsoas signs	i. Peritonitis
_____ 9. Localized infection in the kidney cortex	j. Acute renal failure
_____ 10. Hypertrophy of the muscle of the pylorus	

Case Study

An 18-year-old woman presents with abdominal pain. Listed below are data collected by the examiner during an interview and examination.

<u>INTERVIEW DATA</u>

The patient tells the examiner the pain started yesterday evening and has gotten progressively worse. She describes the pain as "really bad." The pain is constant and located in her right lower abdomen toward her umbilicus. She says that her pain feels a little better if she stays curled up and does not move. She tells the examiner that she is in good health and that she has never had a problem with her stomach. She indicates that normally she has a good appetite and can eat anything. She says she ate breakfast and lunch yesterday, but by dinnertime she was nauseated and had no appetite. She has not eaten anything since. She denies any recent weight changes, but she says she would like to weigh about 5 pounds less than she currently does. She does not smoke or drink alcoholic beverages, and she takes no medication. She denies discomfort or problems with urination, describing her urine as "usual looking."

<u>EXAMINATION DATA</u>

General survey: Alert and anxious young woman in moderate distress lying in a fetal position on the examination table with her eyes closed. Appears well nourished but not obese. Her skin is hot.

Abdominal inspection: Abdomen is flat and symmetric. No lesions or scars noted. No surface movements are seen except for breathing.

Abdominal auscultation: Bowel sounds absent.

Abdominal percussion: Tympany noted over most of abdominal surface; dullness over liver. Midclavicular liver span is 4 inches.

Light abdominal palpation: Demonstrates pain and guarding in right lower quadrant. Unable to palpate deep structures because of excessive abdominal discomfort. Demonstrates positive rebound tenderness in right lower quadrant.

1. What data deviate from normal findings, suggesting a need for further investigation?

2. What additional questions could the examiner ask to clarify symptoms?

3. What additional physical examination, if any, should the examiner complete?

4. What primary problems does the patient have?

CLINICAL REASONING

1. As you auscultate the abdomen, you should listen not only for bowel sounds but also for vascular sounds and a friction rub. List specifically what you are listening to and what abnormal findings may indicate.

2. Your patient is a 46-year-old man with liver cirrhosis. You are preparing to check for ascites using a fluid wave technique. How is this particular procedure done, and what is a positive finding?

3. A 24-year-old woman is 7 months pregnant. Describe expected findings during an abdominal examination that are unique to pregnancy.

Patient Safety Consideration

What precaution would you take when examining the abdomen of a patient with suspected mononucleosis? Why? What related advice might you give the patient if the diagnosis is confirmed?

Multiple Choice

Circle the best answer for each of the following questions.

1. Which statement suggests that a patient may be at risk for contracting viral hepatitis A?
   a. "I am a healthcare worker."
   b. "I had a blood transfusion recently."
   c. "I have renal failure and have hemodialysis three times a week."
   d. "I have recently been overseas."

2. The examiner observes venous return on the abdomen of the patient that moves upward from the pubis to the chest. This finding should make the examiner consider
   a. portal hypertension.
   b. renal artery stenosis.
   c. inferior vena cava obstruction.
   d. mesentery arterial hypertension.

3. A woman who is 36 weeks pregnant tells the examiner that her stomach muscle feels like it is splitting. A protrusion at the midline of the abdomen is observed. This is recognized as
   a. abdominal dehiscence.
   b. swelling of the abdominal aorta.
   c. diastasis recti.
   d. umbilical herniation.

4. In which of the following patients would a slight pulsation in the upper midline of the abdomen be considered a normal inspection finding?
   a. A very thin patient
   b. An obese patient
   c. A patient with ascites
   d. An older patient

5. The examiner palpates an organ in the left costal margin. Which technique should the examiner use to differentiate between an enlarged left kidney and an enlarged spleen?
   a. Auscultation, listening for renal bruit
   b. Auscultation, listening for abdominal friction rub
   c. Palpation, using indirect fist palpation to assess for tenderness
   d. Percussion, listening for dullness

6. A hiatal hernia is best described as
   a. a protrusion of abdominal contents through a weakening in the abdominal wall.
   b. a protrusion of the stomach through the esophageal opening in the diaphragm.
   c. an ulcer in the mucosa of the stomach that herniates into the peritoneal cavity.
   d. a herniation of the gallbladder into the cystic duct.

7. An examiner may wish to use a bimanual technique for abdominal palpation when
   a. palpating superficial organs.
   b. validating abdominal tenderness in the infant.
   c. meeting muscle resistance while performing deep palpation.
   d. determining the presence of excessive peritoneal fluid.

8. A 2½-year-old child presents with abdominal pain and stools that are red currant jelly in appearance. Which problem would the examiner suspect?
   a. Meckel diverticulum
   b. Pyloric stenosis
   c. Intussusception
   d. Necrotizing enterocolitis

9. You note that the midclavicular liver span of an adult male patient is 18 cm. With palpation, you note that the liver is enlarged and nontender. What do these findings suggest?
   a. Diverticulitis
   b. Ulcerative colitis
   c. Hepatitis
   d. Cirrhosis

10. The examiner is unable to palpate a patient's liver. Which of the following techniques will help assess tenderness in this organ?
    a. Application of continuous, firm pressure for 3 to 5 minutes
    b. Percussion for tympany
    c. Percussion for size
    d. Indirect fist percussion

11. Where is pain felt when an obturator muscle test is positive?
    a. Right hip and thigh
    b. Right hypogastric area
    c. Right lower quadrant and groin
    d. Beneath the right shoulder blade

12. Which of the following techniques is used to confirm the presence of abdominal ascites?
    a. Auscultation of fluid movement within the abdominal cavity
    b. Palpation of rebound tenderness
    c. Palpation of pitting edema on the abdomen
    d. Percussion of dullness over dependent areas of the abdomen

13. Which of the following examination findings is indicative of peritoneal irritation or appendicitis?
    a. Rebound tenderness on palpation
    b. Shifting dullness over the abdomen on percussion
    c. Bruit heard over the abdominal aorta on auscultation
    d. Dullness over the suprapubic area on percussion

14. Which finding on a newborn infant suggests a congenital anomaly?
    a. The umbilical cord has one artery and one vein.
    b. The umbilical cord is thick.
    c. The umbilical cord is thin.
    d. There is a small mass around the umbilicus.

15. A 61-year-old man has a presenting complaint of frequent constipation. He tells the examiner that there has been a change in his bowel movement habits—he gets constipated easily, the stool is very "skinny looking," and it is a different color than usual. He denies pain. What do these symptoms suggest?
    a. Diverticulitis
    b. Hepatitis B
    c. Colon or rectal cancer
    d. Pancreatitis

16. The functional ability of the gastrointestinal tract most severely affected by aging is
    a. motility.
    b. metabolism.
    c. digestion.
    d. catabolism.

17. Which rule states that the farther away from the navel abdominal pain occurs, the more likely it is to be of pathological importance?
    a. Reglan rule
    b. Apley rule
    c. Applegate rule
    d. Romberg rule

18. Ecchymosis of the flanks associated with pancreatitis is identified as which of the following signs?
    a. Grey Turner
    b. Aaron
    c. Dance
    d. Markle

19. Which of the following is the correct sequence for examining the abdomen?
    a. Inspection, auscultation, percussion, palpation
    b. Auscultation, inspection, percussion, palpation
    c. Inspection, auscultation, palpation, percussion
    d. Percussion, inspection, auscultation, palpation

20. Which of the following identifies the Murphy sign?
    a. Pain down the medial aspect of the thigh to the knees
    b. Abrupt cessation of inspiration on palpation of the gallbladder
    c. Rebound tenderness and sharp pain when the right lower quadrant is palpated
    d. Right lower quadrant pain intensified by left lower clutching abdominal palpation

21. Peritoneal irritation is associated with which of the following signs?
    a. Aaron
    b. Ballance
    c. Blumberg
    d. Dance

22. Abdominal pain radiating to the left shoulder may be indicative of which of the following?
    a. Appendicitis
    b. Intussusception
    c. Pancreatitis
    d. Splenic rupture

19 Female Genitalia

LEARNING OBJECTIVES

After studying Chapter 19 in the textbook and completing this section of the laboratory manual, students should be able to:

1. Conduct a history related to the female genitalia.
2. Discuss examination techniques for the female genitalia.
3. Identify normal age- and condition-related variations of the female genitalia.
4. Recognize findings that deviate from expected findings.
5. Relate symptoms or clinical findings to common pathologic conditions.

TERMINOLOGY REVIEW

Check your understanding of terminology related to assessment of the female genitalia. Using the space provided, write the word or phrase from the list next to the appropriate descriptor.

Ambiguous genitalia	**Infertility**
Atrophic vaginitis	**Menarche**
Bartholin glands	**Mittelschmerz**
Caruncle	**Rectocele**
Chadwick sign	**Rectouterine pouch**
Cystocele	**Skene ducts**
Hegar sign	**Uterine prolapse**
Hydrocolpos	

1. _____: inflammation of the vagina caused by the thinning and shrinking of tissues, as well as decreased lubrication; caused by a lack of estrogen during perimenopause and menopause.

2. _____: distention of the vagina resulting from an accumulation of fluid caused by congenital vaginal obstruction; obstruction usually caused by an imperforate hymen; or, less commonly, a transverse vaginal septum.

3. _____: a bluish discoloration of the cervix that normally occurs in pregnancy at 8–12 weeks' gestation.

4. _____: a deep recess formed by the peritoneum between the rectum and cervix (cul-de-sac of Douglas).

5. _____: descent or herniation of the uterus into or beyond the vagina; the result of weakening of the supporting structures of the pubic floor.

6. _____: a small, bright-red growth protruding from the urethral meatus; most urethral caruncles do not cause symptoms.

7. _____: the onset of first menstruation, which usually occurs between 12 and 13 years of age.

8. _____: glands located posteriorly on each side of the vaginal orifice, open onto the sides of the vestibule in the groove between the labia minora and the hymen.

9. _____: the inability to conceive over a period of 1 year; contributing factors with women include abnormalities of the vagina, cervix, uterus, fallopian tubes, and ovaries.

10. _____: hernial protrusion of part of the rectum into the vagina.

11. _____: softening of the cervix that is a sign of pregnancy, occurring at 6–8 weeks' gestation.

12. _____: a newborn's genitalia are not clearly either male or female; usually caused by genetic abnormalities.

13. _____: hernial protrusion of the urinary bladder into the vagina, sometimes exiting the introitus.

14. _____: lower abdominal pain associated with ovulation; may be accompanied by tenderness on the side where ovulation took place that month.

15. _____: these drain a group of urethral glands and open into the vestibule on each side of the urethra.

APPLICATION TO CLINICAL PRACTICE

Anatomy Review
Identify the structures of the female anatomy labeled on the illustration by writing the correct term in the blank next to the corresponding letter on the next page.

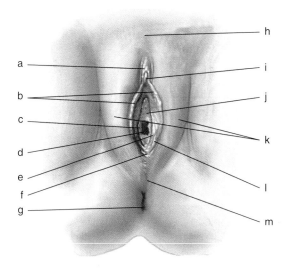

From Lowdermilk DL, Perry SE. *Maternity and Women's Health Care*, 8th ed. St. Louis, MO: Mosby, 2007.

a. _____	Anus
b. _____	Bartholin duct opening
c. _____	Clitoris
d. _____	Fourchette
e. _____	Hymen
f. _____	Labium majus
g. _____	Labium minus
h. _____	Mons pubis
i. _____	Perineum
j. _____	Prepuce
k. _____	Urethral or urinary orifice
l. _____	Vaginal orifice
m. _____	Vestibule

Matching 1

Match each type of malignancy with its corresponding risk factors. Some risk factors apply to more than one malignancy.

Risk Factor	Malignancy
_____ 1. History of breast cancer	O: ovarian cancer
_____ 2. Smoking	C: cervical cancer
_____ 3. Infertility or nulliparity	E: endometrial cancer
_____ 4. Low socioeconomic status	
_____ 5. Multiple pregnancies	
_____ 6. Early menarche + late menopause	
_____ 7. Obesity	
_____ 8. Infection with HPV	

Matching 2

Match each diagnostic laboratory test with the type of instrument used to collect the specimen.

Diagnostic Test	Instrument Used
_____ 1. Gonococcal culture	a. Dacron swab
_____ 2. Endocervical cells	b. KOH prep
_____ 3. DNA probe for chlamydia and gonorrhea	c. Spatula
_____ 4. *Trichomonas vaginalis*	d. Sterile cotton swab
_____ 5. Both ectocervical and endocervical cells	e. Cylindric-type brush
_____ 6. Candidiasis	f. Wet mount
_____ 7. Ectocervical cells	g. Cervical broom

Concepts Application

Listed below are several alternatives to the traditional lithotomy position for pelvic examination. Compare these alternatives by describing each position and listing advantages or disadvantages of each.

Position	Description	Advantages or Disadvantages
Knee–chest		
Diamond shape		
Obstetric stirrups		
M-shape		
V-shape		

Case Study

A 33-year-old woman presents to the urgent care center. Listed below are data collected by the examiner during the interview and examination.

INTERVIEW DATA

The patient tells the examiner, "I have a really bad pain in front of my butt. It hurts so much that I can't even wipe with a tissue after I go to the bathroom." She indicates that the pain started 2 days ago and is much worse now. When asked about her sexual activity, Ms. Harris says, "I have a guy that I'm with, but it's not exclusive or anything. We see other people and try not to be real serious."

EXAMINATION DATA

External: Typical hair distribution; urethral meatus intact; no redness or discharge. Perineum intact. Extreme pain response to palpation of vaginal opening. Swelling, redness, and mass detected on right side. Foul-smelling discharge noted.

Internal: Examination deferred because of extreme pain associated with inflammation.

1. What data deviate from normal findings, suggesting a need for further investigation?

2. What additional questions could the examiner ask to clarify symptoms?

3. What additional physical examination, if any, should the examiner complete?

4. What primary problems does the patient have?

CLINICAL REASONING

1. A 42-year-old blind woman presents for a routine examination. How should the examiner approach this patient to best meet her needs?

2. A 16-year-old girl is in the clinic for a school sports physical. How should her health history and an examination of her genitalia differ from that of an adult?

Patient Safety Consideration

How do you prevent accidental damage to tissues when a vaginal speculum is withdrawn?

CONTENT REVIEW QUESTIONS

Multiple Choice

Circle the best answer for each of the following questions:

1. Which finding is suggestive of pelvic inflammatory disease?
   a. Enlargement of the ovaries
   b. Everted cervix
   c. Tender bilateral adnexal areas
   d. Unilateral labial swelling, redness, and tenderness

2. Which finding would be of concern during an examination of an older female patient?
   a. Palpable ovaries
   b. Small and pale cervix
   c. Constriction of the vaginal introitus
   d. Absence of vaginal rugation

3. While palpating the introitus of the vagina, the patient jumps and complains of severe tenderness. A mass is palpated that is warm to touch. With which of the following problems are these clinical findings consistent?
   a. Cancer of the cervix
   b. Inflammation of the Bartholin glands
   c. A cystocele
   d. Acute genital wart infection

4. Which finding may be indicative of a pelvic mass? The cervix is
   a. pale in color.
   b. deviating to the right.
   c. protruding 2.5 cm into the vagina.
   d. pointing anteriorly.

5. Which finding on inspection of the external genitalia of a nulliparous 72-year-old female would you consider normal?
   a. The urinary meatus appears as an irregular opening.
   b. The clitoris appears prominent and enlarged.
   c. The vaginal introitus appears flaccid and gaping.
   d. Labia appear moist, distended, and dull.

6. A patient complains of pain; dysmenorrhea; and heavy, prolonged menstrual flow. Tender nodules are palpable along the uterosacral ligament. These symptoms and findings suggest
   a. pelvic inflammatory disease.
   b. endometriosis.
   c. ectopic pregnancy.
   d. ovarian cancer.

7. An examiner plans to collect samples for cytologic studies during a vaginal examination. Use of which type of lubricant on the speculum is least likely to interfere with specimen analysis and interpretation?
   a. A water-soluble lubricant
   b. Topical anesthetizing ointment
   c. Warm water
   d. Vaginal secretions

8. Symptoms associated with premenstrual syndrome (PMS) are caused by
   a. ovulation.
   b. thickening of the uterine lining.
   c. elevations in body temperature.
   d. fluctuations in hormone levels.

9. When examining a middle-aged woman with a history of endometrial cancer and a hysterectomy, the examiner should
   a. avoid the bimanual and palpation maneuvers.
   b. obtain a Pap smear from the suture line.
   c. omit cultures and specimens from the vagina.
   d. palpate internal areas before inserting the speculum.

10. A patient complains of urinary incontinence when she is active. Which associated finding might explain this problem?
    a. Herniation of the rectum into the posterior vaginal wall
    b. Presence of a cystocele.
    c. History of PMS
    d. Protrusion of an enlarged cervix into the vaginal vault

11. Which finding suggests a sexually transmitted infection?
    a. Ulcers and vesicles on the vulva
    b. Atrophy of labia minora
    c. Dilation of the urethral orifice
    d. Bluish color to the cervix

12. The examiner observes a slit-shaped cervical os in a nulliparous woman. Which of the following data in her history explains this finding? The patient
    a. had an early onset of menarche.
    b. has had multiple sex partners.
    c. has had infection with the HPV.
    d. had an abortion as a teenager.

13. A prominent labia minora in a newborn
    a. indicates a maternal infection.
    b. suggests ambiguous genitalia.
    c. is consistent with prematurity.
    d. is a normal finding.

14. Softness of the cervix is an expected finding for
    a. an adolescent.
    b. a pregnant woman.
    c. a nonpregnant woman.
    d. an older adult.

15. By which week of pregnancy would you expect to be able to palpate the uterus at the symphysis pubis?
    a. 8th
    b. 10th
    c. 12th
    d. 14th

16. A cauliflower-like mass found on the labia of a female patient is most likely caused by
    a. primary syphilis.
    b. condyloma latum.
    c. condyloma acuminatum.
    d. venereal herpes.

17. A sexually active, single, 22-year-old patient complains of a "gross" vaginal discharge. Which of the following questions would help the examiner understand this symptom?
    a. "Do you use condoms?"
    b. "What type of oral contraceptives do you take?"
    c. "At what age did you start menstruating?"
    d. "Do you have a family history of ovarian or breast cancer?"

18. A 62-year-old female patient went through menopause about 14 years ago. Which statement made by this patient indicates a need for further follow-up?
    a. "I have not been sexually active for about 4 years."
    b. "My pubic hair has become very thin."
    c. "I have small amounts of vaginal bleeding a couple of times a week."
    d. "I have been taking extra calcium since I reached menopause."

19. A patient reports that, over the past year, the interval between her menstrual periods has lengthened and her last three periods have been about 6 weeks apart. Which term describes this problem?
    a. Amenorrhea
    b. Hypomenorrhea
    c. Hypermenorrhea
    d. Oligomenorrhea

20. Which is an additional piece of information that you would include on the lab requisition if a cervical Pap smear has been obtained from a transgender man?
    a. Gender genotype
    b. Years since change in gender identity
    c. Use of testosterone
    d. Number and gender of sexual partners

20 Male Genitalia

LEARNING OBJECTIVES

After studying Chapter 20 in the textbook and completing this section of the laboratory manual, students should be able to:
1. Conduct a history related to the male genitalia.
2. Discuss examination techniques for the male genitalia.
3. Identify normal age- and condition-related variations of the male genitalia.
4. Recognize findings that deviate from expected findings.
5. Relate symptoms and clinical findings to common pathologic conditions.

TERMINOLOGY REVIEW

Check your understanding of terminology related to assessment of the male genitalia. Using the space provided, write the word or phrase from the list next to the appropriate descriptor.

Adhesions	**Hypospadias**
Chordee	**Peyronie**
Cremasteric	**Phimosis or paraphimosis**
Cryptorchidism	**Priapism**
Escutcheon	**Spermatocele**
Glans	**Testicular torsion**
Hydrocele	**Varicocele**

1. _____: the inability to replace the foreskin to its usual position after it has been retracted behind the glands.

2. _____: ventral shortening and curvature of the penis.

3. _____: benign cystic accumulation of sperm on the epididymis.

4. _____: expansion at the distal end of the penis by the corpus spongiosum.

5. _____: prolonged penile erection.

6. _____: fluid accumulation in the scrotum as a result of a defect in the tunica vaginalis, resulting in a nontender, smooth, and firm mass.

7. _____: inflammatory bands that connect opposing serous surfaces.

8. _____: pattern of hair growth on the male pubis and abdomen.

9. _____: rotation producing ischemia of the testis.

10. _____: abnormal tortuosity and dilation of veins of the pampiniform plexus in the spermatic cord.

11. _____: undescended testes; a scrotum that has remained small, flat, and undeveloped.

12. _____: reflex characterized by rising of the scrotum and testicle when the inner thigh is stroked.

13. _____: congenital defect in which the urethral meatus is located on the ventral surface of the glans penile shaft or the base of the penis.

14. _____: disease characterized by a fibrous band in the corpus cavernosum.

Anatomy Review

Identify the structures of the male anatomy labeled on the illustration below by writing the correct term in the blank next to the corresponding letter on the next page. Use each term once.

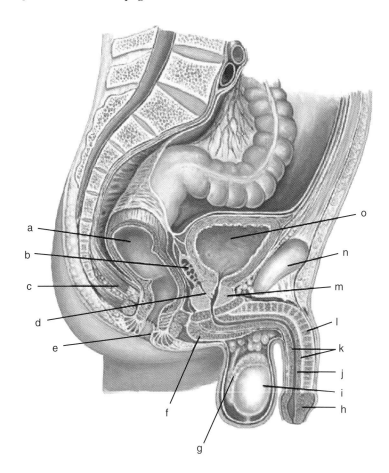

a. _____	Anus
b. _____	Bulbocavernosus muscle
c. _____	Corpus cavernosum
d. _____	Corpus spongiosum
e. _____	Ejaculatory duct
f. _____	Epididymis
g. _____	Glans
h. _____	Levator ani muscle
i. _____	Prostate gland
j. _____	Rectum
k. _____	Seminal vesicle
l. _____	Symphysis pubis
m. _____	Testis
n. _____	Urethra
o. _____	Urinary bladder

Matching 1

Match each lesion description with the corresponding sexually transmitted infection.

Description of Lesion	Sexually Transmitted Infection
____ 1. Initially, a painless erosion on or near the coronal sulcus	a. Syphilitic chancre
____ 2. Painful superficial vesicles on the glans, penile shaft, or base of the penis	b. Genital herpes
____ 3. Dome-shaped, smooth, pearly gray lesions on the glans penis	c. Genital warts
____ 4. Painless lesion with a clear base and indurated borders, usually located on the glans penis	d. Lymphogranuloma venereum
____ 5. Reddish lesions on the prepuce, glans, and shaft; may also be present within the urethra	e. Molluscum contagiosum

Match each examination technique with its corresponding purpose.

Examination Technique	Purpose
_____ 1. Foreskin retracted	a. Inspecting for urethral discharge
_____ 2. Finger moved along vas deferens	b. Observing for hydrocele
_____ 3. Glans pressed between thumb and forefinger	c. Observing for phimosis
_____ 4. Mass transilluminated	d. Palpating for inguinal hernia
_____ 5. Testes gently compressed	e. Palpating for tender testes

Case Study

A 43-year-old man presents to the urgent care center. Listed below are data collected by the examiner.

INTERVIEW DATA

The patient tells the examiner, "Yesterday I noticed a mild discomfort in my groin. When I looked, I saw this area of swelling." The examiner asks about recent activity. The patient replies, "We have been in the process of moving, and I have been picking up heavy boxes, moving furniture, and climbing up and down ladders all weekend."

EXAMINATION DATA

General survey: Healthy-appearing man.

Examination: Bulge noted in area of Hesselbach triangle that is painless. Inguinal area on right side with a palpable mass. Pushes against side of finger on examination.

1. What data deviate from normal findings, suggesting a need for further investigation?

2. What additional questions could the examiner ask to clarify symptoms?

3. What additional physical examination, if any, should the examiner complete?

4. What primary problems does the patient have?

CLINICAL REASONING

1. A 30-year-old man requests information regarding self-examination of his genitalia. What information should the examiner share with him?

2. When the examiner attempts to examine the genitalia of a 5-year-old boy, the boy refuses to take off his pants and says, "You can't see my privates." What measures can the examiner take to facilitate this part of the examination?

Patient Safety Consideration

Why do you not force the retraction of the foreskin when examining the genitals of an infant or young child?

Multiple Choice

Circle the best answer for each of the following questions:

1. While examining a newborn male infant, the examiner palpates a testicle in the inguinal canal that cannot be pushed into the scrotum. This finding is consistent with
   a. a retractile testis.
   b. ambiguous genitalia.
   c. a direct inguinal hernia.
   d. an undescended testicle.

2. Genital self-examination (GSE) should be taught to patients who are at risk for
   a. testicular cancer.
   b. Peyronie disease.
   c. sexually transmitted infection.
   d. prostate enlargement.

3. On examination of a patient's scrotum, you note that it is unusually thickened and it pits. What is one type of problem suggested by these findings?
   a. Sexually transmitted disease
   b. Squamous cell skin cancer
   c. Liver disease
   d. Autoimmune disease

4. While examining the genitalia of a 2-year-old boy, the examiner should be aware that the
   a. scrotum is normally edematous until age 4 years.
   b. foreskin of the uncircumcised penis is not fully re-tractable until age 3 or 4 years.
   c. testicles typically do not descend into the scrotum until age 5 years.
   d. cremasteric reflex does not become evident until age 6 or 7.

5. Which item in the patient history is considered a risk factor for cancer of the penis?
   a. Circumcised at birth
   b. History of condyloma acuminatum infections
   c. Had a congenital hydrocele
   d. History of untreated epispadias

6. In which of the following situations is transillumina-tion of the scrotum indicated?
   a. Presence of syphilis chancre is noted.
   b. Indirect hernia is palpated.
   c. The examiner suspects a mass.
   d. The examiner palpates the testes.

7. The patient is asked to bear down while the examiner palpates the inguinal ring. The examiner feels a soft swelling sensation on the fingertip. The patient com-plains of pain while straining. These findings are consistent with which of the following?
   a. Indirect hernia
   b. Direct hernia
   c. Femoral hernia
   d. Rectal hernia

8. The examiner inspects the scrotum of a 43-year-old man. Which finding requires further evaluation or follow-up?
   a. The left testicle hangs lower than the right testicle.
   b. The scrotum is darker than the general skin color.
   c. The skin on the scrotum is shiny and smooth.
   d. The scrotum has a midline raphe.

9. Which finding may indicate diabetes?
   a. The vas deferens feels beaded or lumpy.
   b. The testicle feels hard with a lump.
   c. Sebaceous cysts are present on the scrotal skin.
   d. The urethra has a slitlike orifice.

10. During an examination for a hernia, an adult male patient should
    a. be asked to stand.
    b. be in a supine position.
    c. sit on a table with the heels together.
    d. assume a knee–chest position on the examination table.

11. Which of the following testicular characteristics is (are) associated with syphilis or diabetic neuropathy?
    a. Asymmetry and drooping
    b. Bilateral enlargement
    c. Insensitivity to pain
    d. Migration into the abdomen

12. What type of hernia would you most likely see in a 15-year-old male?
    a. Femoral hernia
    b. Umbilical hernia
    c. Direct inguinal hernia
    d. Indirect inguinal hernia

13. Which patient characteristic is associated with smegma as an expected finding?
    a. Uncircumcised
    b. Prepubertal
    c. Sexually active
    d. Transgender

14. A 24-year-old man has scrotal pain and marked erythema. The examiner considers epididymitis. Which other finding is most consistent with this problem?
    a. Absent cremasteric reflex
    b. Anorexia and nausea
    c. Acute onset of severe pain
    d. Urethral discharge

15. Hypospadias is a congenital defect in which the urethra meatus is located on the ventral surface of the glans penis. This is thought to occur embryologically during urethral development during which stage of gestation?
    a. 4–6 weeks
    b. 8–20 weeks
    c. 15–25 weeks
    d. 20–30 weeks

16. Which of the following hernias occurs more often in females and is the least common of all hernias?
    a. Indirect
    b. Direct
    c. Femoral
    d. Ventral

17. Which finding on examination of a scrotal mass, which is neither a testicle or spermatic cord, suggests the problem is an incarcerated hernia?
    a. The mass does not transilluminate nor change in size when reduction is attempted.
    b. The mass does not transilluminate but decreases in size when reduction is attempted.
    c. The mass transilluminates but does not change in size when reduction is attempted.
    d. The mass both transilluminates and changes in size when reduction is attempted.

18. You examine a 22-year-old patient. His chief complaint is penile pain and swelling. On examination, you note a constricting band of tissue directly behind the head of the penis. You diagnose this as
    a. paraphimosis.
    b. hypospadias.
    c. orchitis.
    d. torsion.

19. You are examining a patient and note pearly-gray, smooth, and umbilicated lesions. The most common cause of these lesions is
    a. syphilis.
    b. condyloma acuminata.
    c. molluscum contagiosum.
    d. lymphogranuloma venereum.

20. Which finding indicates a normal cremasteric reflex?
    a. Penile erection in response to light touch
    b. Descent of a testicle into the scrotum in response to pressure on the abdominal wall.
    c. Drop of urine appearing at the urethral meatus in response to pressing the glans.
    d. Elevation of the left testicle and scrotum in response to stroking the left inner thigh.

Anus, Rectum, and Prostate

After studying Chapter 21 in the textbook and completing this section of the laboratory manual, students should be able to:
1. Conduct a history related to the anus, rectum, and prostate.
2. Discuss examination techniques for the anus, rectum, and prostate.
3. Identify normal age- and condition-related variations of the anus, rectum, and prostate.
4. Recognize findings that deviate from expected findings.
5. Relate symptoms and clinical findings to common pathologic conditions.

TERMINOLOGY REVIEW

Check your understanding of terminology related to assessment of the anus, rectum, and prostate. Using the space provided, write the word or phrase from the list next to the appropriate descriptor.

Anal canal	**Pilonidal cyst**
Anal fistula	**Polyp**
Anorectal fissure	**Prostate**
Enterobiasis (roundworm or pinworm)	**Pruritus ani**
Hemorrhoids	**Rectal prolapse**
Imperforate anus	**Rectum**

1. _____: a gland located at the base of the bladder and surrounding the urethra; it is composed of muscular and glandular tissue.

2. _____: varicose veins in the rectum that may be external below the anorectal line or internal above the anorectal line; caused by pressure on the veins in the pelvic and rectal areas from straining, diarrhea, constipation, or prolonged sitting.

3. _____: inflammatory tract that runs from the anus or rectum and opens onto the surface of the perianal skin or other tissue; caused by inflammation from a perianal or perirectal abscess.

4. _____: the terminal portion of the gastrointestinal tract.

5. _____: a congenital defect in which the rectal opening is blocked or missing; one of a variety of anorectal malformations that can occur during fetal development.

6. _____: infection caused by a small, thin, white roundworm (*Enterobius vermicularis*) adult nematode (parasite) that lives in the rectum or colon and emerges onto the perianal skin to lay eggs while the person sleeps; common in children.

7. _____: itching of the anal area; commonly caused by fungal infection in adults and by parasites in children.

8. _____: terminal portion of the rectum; lined by columns of mucosal tissue (columns of Morgagni), that fuse to form the anorectal junction.

9. _____: condition in which the rectal mucosa (with or without the muscular wall) protrudes through the anal ring; results from constipation, diarrhea, or sometimes severe coughing or straining.

10. _____: a cyst or sinus near the cleft of the buttocks; excessive pressure or repetitive trauma to the sacrococcygeal area predisposes individuals to the development of the cyst.

117

11. _____: a tear in the anal mucosa; appears most often in the posterior midline as a result of posttraumatic passage of large hard stools.

12. _____: abnormal growth of tissue projecting from the mucous membrane; may occur anywhere in the intestinal tract and be malignant or benign.

Anatomy Review 1

Identify the structures of the rectum labeled on the illustration by writing the correct term in the blank next to the corresponding letter.

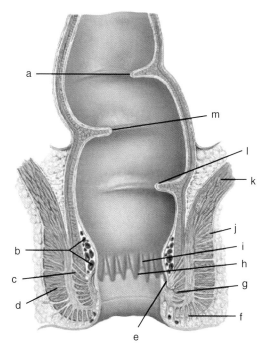

a. _____	Anal crypt
b. _____	Deep external sphincter
c. _____	Inferior rectal valve
d. _____	Internal hemorrhoidal plexus
e. _____	Internal sphincter
f. _____	Levator ani muscle
g. _____	Middle rectal valve
h. _____	Perianal gland
i. _____	Rectal column
j. _____	Rectal sinus
k. _____	Subcutaneous external sphincter
l. _____	Superficial external sphincter
m. _____	Superior rectal valve

Anatomy Review 2

Identify the structures of the prostate labeled on the illustration by writing the correct term in the blank next to the corresponding letter.

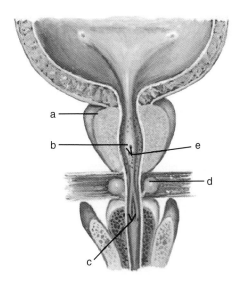

a.	_____	Cowper gland
b.	_____	Ejaculatory orifice
c.	_____	Opening of Cowper gland
d.	_____	Prostate gland
e.	_____	Utricle

Matching

Match each examination finding or symptom with the corresponding problem to be considered.

Examination finding or symptom	Problem
_____ 1. Severe rectal pain with a fever	a. Prostatitis
_____ 2. Absence of meconium stool passage in an infant	b. Perianal abscess
_____ 3. Feels smooth and firm with a 4-cm protrusion into the rectum	c. Rectal polyp
_____ 4. Elevated red granular tissue opening on perianal skin	d. Benign prostatic hypertrophy
_____ 5. Feels enlarged, asymmetric, and tender to palpation	e. Prostatic carcinoma
_____ 6. Feels hard, nodular; unable to palpate sulcus	f. Imperforate anus
_____ 7. Soft nodules palpated with rectal examination	g. Anorectal fistula

Case Study

A 66-year-old man presents to his primary care provider because of a persistent feeling of rectal fullness over the past 3 months. Listed below are data collected by the examiner during an interview and examination.

Interview Data

The patient tells the examiner he has had pain "off and on" but became concerned when he started seeing blood in his stool. The blood is described as "bright red." He also states that he has seen spots on his underwear, but he has ignored it, thinking he had hemorrhoids. When asked about changes in his diet, he indicates that he really hasn't been very hungry lately and has lost 10 pounds over the past several months.

Examination Data

General survey: Thin-appearing man. Vital signs are within normal limits.

Rectal examination: Perineal and anal inspection is unremarkable with no lesions, dimpling, or changes in skin characteristics. Sphincter tone findings unremarkable. A large mass is felt with rectal palpation extending from the posterior to the left lateral rectal wall. The prostate is smooth, firm, and nontender to palpation, with a 1-cm protrusion.

1. What data deviate from normal findings, suggesting a need for further investigation?

2. What additional questions could the examiner ask to clarify symptoms?

3. What additional physical examination, if any, should the examiner complete?

4. What primary problems does the patient have?

CLINICAL REASONING

1. A 68-year-old man comes to the emergency department with a history of urinary retention. He states, "I know my bladder is full, but I can't seem to pee." This symptom could be caused by prostatitis, benign prostate hypertrophy, or prostatic carcinoma. How does the examiner differentiate the cause of this patient's symptom?

2. A 70-year-old woman comes to a clinic with a complaint of rectal bleeding. There are multiple causes of rectal bleeding. What kind of interview questions should be asked to help the examiner narrow down the cause of the problem?

Patient Safety Consideration

When examining the position and patency of a neonate's anus, care must be taken not to confuse a _____ with an anal orifice.

CONTENT REVIEW QUESTIONS

Multiple Choice

Circle the best answer for each of the following questions:

1. While palpating the lateral and posterior rectal walls, the examiner should expect to palpate
   a. a smooth, even, and uninterrupted surface.
   b. small nodules from internal hemorrhoids.
   c. tissue folds from the valves of Houston.
   d. bulging from the bladder wall.

2. A patient presents with a chief complaint of rectal pain. The examiner will focus the history and examination on which known fact?
   a. Rectal pain is almost always accompanied by an infection.
   b. Rectal pain is almost always an indication of local disease.
   c. A complaint of rectal pain is usually associated with a serious systemic process.
   d. One of the most common causes of rectal pain is prostatic enlargement.

3. Which is an appropriate response when a transwoman patient who had a gonadectomy says "I am very glad I don't have to worry about prostate cancer anymore."?
   a. "That is definitely a benefit of the surgery."
   b. "Your risk for prostate cancer may be reduced but it is not eliminated."
   c. "Your risk for prostate cancer is lowered but not eliminated."
   d. "Unfortunately, the surgery actually increases your risk to a slight degree."

4. While examining the perineum of a 6-year-old girl, the examiner observes hemorrhoids. This finding suggests
   a. repeated events of sexual abuse.
   b. the presence of chronic constipation.
   c. a diet high in fibrous foods.
   d. an underlying problem, such as portal hypertension.

5. To examine a prostate, what surface is palpated?
   a. Anterior rectal wall surface
   b. Posterior rectal wall surface
   c. Anterior prostate surface
   d. Deep external sphincter surface

6. A patient has fatty stools. Which problems are suggested by this finding?
   a. pancreatic disorders, malabsorption syndromes
   b. tropical sprue, carcinoma of the hepatopancreatic ampulla
   c. Crohn disease, amebiasis
   d. Ulcerative colitis, diverticulitis.

7. An older male patient is unable to assume a standing position for a routine rectal examination. What is the best alternative position?
   a. Lithotomy position
   b. Left lateral position with the knees flexed
   c. Knee–chest position
   d. Prone position

8. A pregnant woman presents to the emergency department with a complaint of dark stools. She tells the examiner, "I read in a magazine that this is a sign of bleeding." Which of the following questions by the examiner is most applicable for this situation?
   a. "Where did you read that information?"
   b. "Have you been giving yourself enemas?"
   c. "How much fruit and vegetable intake have you had in the past few days?"
   d. "Are you taking prenatal vitamins or supplements?"

9. Before palpating the prostate, the examiner should tell the patient that he might feel the urge to do which of the following?
   a. Urinate
   b. Defecate
   c. Vomit
   d. Faint

10. Which behavior observed while you are obtaining a history on a new patient to the clinic is most suggestive of a very acute rectal problem?
    a. Rapidly tapping the feet up and down
    b. Repeatedly crossing and uncrossing the legs
    c. Constant shifting side to side in the chair
    d. Slowly rubbing a hip and thigh

11. Which examination finding in the child is a clue to the diagnosis of Hirschsprung disease?
    a. Passing of frequent, loose stools in the absence of other symptoms
    b. Consistently empty rectum with a history of constipation
    c. Itching and irritation around the anus
    d. Rectal prolapse

12. In which situation would the examiner perform a rectal examination on an infant or child?
    a. A newborn infant passes a greenish-black, viscous stool 12 hours after birth.
    b. The mother of a 3-month-old baby describes the baby's stools as "loose and golden yellow."
    c. A stool of a 6-year-old child is guaiac positive.
    d. A mother tells the examiner that her 3-year-old child was sent home from daycare after two episodes of diarrhea.

13. How is the anal ring assessed?
    a. Inspection of the anus
    b. External palpation of the anus
    c. Examination of the stool
    d. Rotation of a finger within the anal sphincter

14. Which of the following best describes the feel of a normal prostate gland?
    a. Soft olive or grape
    b. Small sea sponge
    c. Ping-pong ball
    d. Pencil eraser

15. Anal patency is verified in a newborn infant by
    a. inserting a lubricated thermometer through the anus and into the rectum.
    b. inserting the fifth digit through the anus and into the rectum.
    c. assessing for the passage of a meconium stool in the first 24–48 hours after birth.
    d. inspecting the anus for an anal opening.

16. Prostate enlargement is determined by the
    a. diameter of the rectum near the bladder.
    b. circumference of the prostate.
    c. estimation of the depth of the sulcus.
    d. protrusion of the prostate into the rectum.

17. Which is the normal response to lightly touching the anal opening?
    a. Dilation of the anus
    b. Contraction of the anal sphincter
    c. Relaxation of the internal sphincter
    d. Shrinking of external hemorrhoids

18. Which direction would you give a patient in order to facilitate visualization of an anal fissure?
    a. "Take a deep breath and hold it."
    b. "Squeeze your buttock muscles."
    c. "Bear down like you're going to have a bowel movement."
    d. "Tighten your muscles as though to stop your flow of urine."

19. The examiner palpates a prostate, noting that it is hard and irregular. The median sulcus is not palpable. These findings are consistent with
    a. prostate cancer.
    b. benign prostatic hypertrophy.
    c. prostatitis.
    d. a rectal mass.

20. A rectal prolapse in a young child is frequently associated with
    a. rickets.
    b. cystic fibrosis.
    c. Crohn disease.
    d. chronic constipation or diarrhea.

22 Musculoskeletal System

LEARNING OBJECTIVES

After studying Chapter 22 in the textbook and completing this section of the laboratory manual, students should be able to:
1. Conduct a history related to the musculoskeletal system.
2. Discuss examination techniques for the musculoskeletal system.
3. Identify normal age- and condition-related variations of the musculoskeletal system.
4. Recognize findings that deviate from expected findings.
5. Relate symptoms and clinical findings to common pathologic conditions.

TERMINOLOGY REVIEW

Check your understanding of terminology related to assessment of the musculoskeletal system. Using the space provided, write the word or phrase from the list next to the appropriate descriptor.

Abduction   Inversion
Adduction   Kyphosis
Crepitus   Muscle strain
Dislocation   Polydactyly
Dupuytren contracture   Pronation
Eversion   Scoliosis
Gibbus   Supination
Goniometer   Syndactyly
Gower sign

1. _____: position of the forearm so that the palm faces down; position of the heel so that the foot does not bear weight through the midline.

2. _____: a condition marked by an abnormal curvature of the spine; the spine may look more like an S or a C.

3. _____: complete separation of the contact between two bones in a joint; caused by pressure or force pushing the bone out of the joint; usually occurs in the setting of acute trauma.

4. _____: movement of the sole of the foot inward at the ankle.

5. _____: excessive stretching or forceful contraction of a muscle beyond its functional capacity.

6. _____: movement of the sole of the foot outward at the ankle.

7. _____: movement of the extremities toward the body.

8. _____: position of the forearm so that the palm faces upward.

9. _____: contractures involving the flexor hand tendons; flexor tendons generally of the fourth and fifth digits contract, causing the fingers to curl with impaired extension.

10. _____: a sign that indicates generalized muscle weakness in children.

11. _____: the presence of more than five digits on the hand or foot.

12. _____: a sharp, angular deformity associated with a collapsed vertebra caused by osteoporosis.

13. _____: a calibrated device designed to measure the arc or range of motion (ROM) of a joint.

14. _____: movement of the extremities away from the body.

15. _____: crackling or grating sound heard in the patient's joint with movement.

16. _____: outward curvature of the thoracic spine.

17. _____: congenital fusion of the digits of the hand or foot.

APPLICATION TO CLINICAL PRACTICE

Matching 1

Match each examination technique with the problem or condition it is used to detect. Some answers may be used more than once.

Examination Technique	Possible Problem or Condition
_____ 1. McMurray test	a. Anterior cruciate ligament injury
_____ 2. Ballottement	b. Effusion of fluid in the knee
_____ 3. Barlow-Ortolani maneuver	c. Flexion contractures in the hip
_____ 4. Bulge sign	d. L1, L2, L3, L4 nerve root irritation
_____ 5. Drawer test	e. Torn meniscus in knee
_____ 6. Femoral stretch test	f. Anteroposterior instability in knee
_____ 7. Lachman test	g. Rotator cuff tear
_____ 8. Neer test	h. Hip subluxation
_____ 9. Thomas test	
_____ 10. Varus/valgus stress test	

Concepts Application 1

Based on the symptoms and/or examination findings provided, list the corresponding problem(s) to consider.

Symptoms or Assessment Findings	Problems to Consider
Heberden nodes and Bouchard nodes noted on the hands	
Low back pain that radiates to the buttocks and posterior thigh with tenderness over the spine	
Heat, redness, swelling, and tenderness to the metatarsophalangeal joint	
Subcutaneous nodules on the forearm near the elbow	
Tenderness, swelling, and boggy sensation with palpation along the grooves of the olecranon process; increased pain with pronation and supination	
A child with muscle atrophy and symptoms of progressive muscle weakness	
A child complaining of pain in the elbow and wrist; will not move his or her arm; maintains arm in a flexed and pronated position	

Match each set of clinical findings with its corresponding diagnosis.

Clinical Findings	Diagnosis
_____ 1. Chronic inflammatory disease involving the spine and sacroiliac joints	a. Bursitis
_____ 2. Numbness, burning, and tingling in the hands	b. Carpal tunnel syndrome
_____ 3. Unilateral facial pain that worsens with joint movement	c. Paget disease
_____ 4. Sudden onset of hot, swollen joint(s), limited ROM	d. Lumbar stenosis
_____ 5. Excessive bone resorption and bone formation	e. Legg-Calvé-Perthes disease
_____ 6. Narrowing of the spinal canal	f. Ankylosing spondylitis
_____ 7. Inflammation of this structure adjacent to a joint leads to limitation with motion, point tenderness, and swelling	g. Temporomandibular joint syndrome
_____ 8. Avascular necrosis of the femoral head	h. Gout

Case Study

The patient is a 46-year-old woman with RA. Listed below are data collected by the examiner during an interview and examination.

INTERVIEW DATA

According to the medical record, the patient was diagnosed with RA at the age of 30 years. She describes a great deal of pain in her joints, particularly in her hands, and says she has just learned to live with the pain because it will always be there. She states that the stiffness and pain in her joints are always worse in the morning or any time she sits around too much. She denies muscle weakness other than the fact that her stiffness and soreness prevent her from doing much. She states that the RA is progressing to the point where she is having difficulty doing things that require fine motor dexterity, such as changing clothes, holding utensils to eat, and cutting up her food. She says she can still get cleaned up but that she had to have different faucet handles installed in her home so she could turn the water on and off. She says she rarely goes out because she feels ugly.

EXAMINATION DATA

Patient is able to stand, but standing up straight and erect is not possible. Gait is slow and purposeful, with jerky movements. Significant inflammation, swelling, and tenderness are noted with inspection and palpation at the hip, knee, wrists, hands, and feet bilaterally. Subcutaneous nodules are noted at ulnar surface of elbows bilaterally.

1. What data deviate from normal findings, suggesting a need for further investigation?

2. What additional questions could the examiner ask to clarify symptoms?

3. What additional physical examination, if any, should the examiner complete?

4. What primary problems does the patient have?

CLINICAL REASONING

1. A 17-year-old male presents with pain in the ankle. He says he twisted it during a soccer game earlier in the afternoon, and now the pain seems to be getting worse. The ankle is very swollen, with a bluish discoloration. How can the examiner differentiate among muscle strain, sprain, or fracture?

2. A 2-year-old girl with a dislocation of the radial head is brought to the clinic by her parents. What type of activities could cause such an injury, and what type of teaching should be provided to the parents?

Patient Safety Consideration

Think about safety and the patient with a musculoskeletal problem. Are the safety needs different for this group of patients than for other patients? Summarize your thoughts.

CONTENT REVIEW QUESTIONS

Multiple Choice

Circle the best answer for each of the following questions:

1. The spine of a newborn infant should be palpated, with the examiner noting the shape of each spinal process. If a split is noted in one of the spinal processes, which problem is suspected?
   a. Bifid defect
   b. Paget disease
   c. Down syndrome
   d. Legg-Calvé-Perthes disease

2. Which of the following questions asked by the examiner would be most helpful in understanding a patient complaining of acute back pain?
   a. "What medications do you currently take?"
   b. "Was there any activity or injury that occurred before the onset of the pain?"
   c. "Were you born with any congenital deformities of the spine?"
   d. "Have you recently lost weight?"

3. Which of the following is commonly seen in a 72-year-old patient?
   a. Meningocele
   b. Myelomeningocele
   c. Kyphosis
   d. Scoliosis

4. Which of the following data from a patient's history indicates an increased risk for osteomyelitis?
   a. Severe gout
   b. Rheumatoid arthritis
   c. Severe osteoporosis
   d. Open fracture of the radius

5. What degree of knee flexion is considered a normal finding?
   a. 15
   b. 90
   c. 130
   d. 160

6. Which of the following is considered a normal finding for a woman in her eighth month of pregnancy?
   a. Stronger ligaments and spinal joints
   b. Hypercalcemia
   c. A 25% loss of muscle strength
   d. Lordosis

7. When assessing for carpal tunnel syndrome, the Tinel sign can be tested by tapping the
   a. dorsal aspect of the wrist.
   b. volar carpal ligament.
   c. radial artery.
   d. median nerve.

8. Which group is susceptible to subluxation of the head of the radius?
   a. Infants and toddlers
   b. Adolescents
   c. Pregnant women
   d. Older adults

9. A patient complains of pain and a clicking noise with jaw movement. The pain extends into the face. These symptoms are suggestive of what condition?
   a. Gout in the jaw
   b. Temporomandibular joint dysfunction
   c. Rheumatoid arthritis of the jaw
   d. Bursitis of the temporomandibular joint

10. "Normal" muscle strength is documented as grade
    a. 0.
    b. 1.
    c. 5.
    d. 10.

11. To assess muscle strength of the temporalis and masseter muscles, the examiner will ask the patient to
    a. push the jaw forward while the examiner applies counterforce.
    b. attempt to open the mouth while the examiner applies counterforce.
    c. clench the teeth while the examiner palpates the contracted muscles.
    d. clench the teeth while the examiner attempts to open the mouth with a tongue blade.

12. For which type of problem does a family history have significance?
    a. Ankylosing spondylitis
    b. Dislocation of radius
    c. Lumbosacral radiculopathy
    d. Bursitis

13. Which statement made by a patient helps the examiner differentiate osteoarthritis from RA?
    a. "I have swelling and pain in my joints."
    b. "I notice a crackling sound when I move my joints."
    c. "I get extremely tired by mid-morning, even when I sleep well."
    d. "I used to play the piano when I was younger."

14. Which of the following would be assessed as part of ROM during the assessment of the thoracic and lumbar spine?
    a. Extension, flexion, and rotation
    b. Eversion, inversion, and rotation
    c. Adduction and abduction
    d. Extension, flexion, and supination

15. A 48-year-old patient presents for the examination of his knee. On examination, you note excessive hyperextension of his knee on weight bearing. This may indicate
    a. genu valgum.
    b. weakness in the quadriceps muscle.
    c. weakness in the cruciate ligament.
    d. weakness in the collateral ligament.

16. A lateral curvature of the thoracic spine indicates
    a. gibbus.
    b. convex curves.
    c. lordosis.
    d. scoliosis.

17. Which of the following tests would detect a torn meniscus?
    a. Ballottement
    b. Varus stress
    c. McMurray
    d. Bulge sign

18. A 28-year-old patient who is in her last trimester of pregnancy presents to your office with complaints of numbness in her left hand. You diagnose her with carpel tunnel syndrome most likely related to
    a. repetitive movement.
    b. fluid retention.
    c. postural changes in the neck caused by pregnancy.
    d. eclampsia.

19. On examination of a patient, you note a difference in size of the upper extremities. You decide that measurement of the circumference is indicated. How do you ensure that the measurements of the two extremities are comparable?
   a. Measure both extremities in centimeters.
   b. Measure at the same distance from the same major landmark.
   c. Measure each extremity twice and average the results for each.
   d. Measure three locations on each extremity and obtain the average.

20. A patient comes to the clinic because of pain and swelling of the proximal interphalangeal joint of the third finger of the left hand. How would you order your examination of her joints?
   a. Affected joint first followed by the same joint on the right hand for comparison.
   b. Left metacarpophalangeal joints, then the left proximal interphalangeal joints, and, finally, the left distal interphalangeal joints.
   c. Affected joint last to avoid inducing discomfort, which could influence the remaining examination.
   d. Left proximal interphalangeal joints starting with the index finger, then the middle finger, then the ring finger, and ending with the fifth finger.

23 Neurologic System

LEARNING OBJECTIVES

After studying Chapter 23 in the textbook and completing this section of the laboratory manual, students should be able to:
1. Conduct a history related to the neurologic system.
2. Discuss examination techniques for the neurologic system.
3. Identify normal age- and condition-related variations of the neurologic system.
4. Recognize findings that deviate from expected findings.
5. Relate symptoms and clinical findings to common pathologic conditions.

TERMINOLOGY REVIEW

Check your understanding of terminology related to assessment of the nervous system. Using the space provided, write the word or phrase from the list next to the appropriate descriptor.

Antalgic	Medulla oblongata
Ataxia	Normal-pressure hydrocephalus
Basal ganglia	Nuchal rigidity
Brainstem	Pseudotumor cerebri
Brudzinski sign	Romberg sign
Cerebellum	Shaken baby syndrome
Frontal lobe	Steppage gait
Graphesthesia	Stereognosis
Hypothalamus	Temporal lobe
Kernig sign	Thalamus
Lower motor neuron disorder	

1. _____: absence of deep tendon reflexes may be an indication of this type of neuron disorder or of peripheral neuropathy.

2. _____: a sign assessed by flexing the leg at the knee and hip and then attempting to straighten the leg of a supine patient.

3. _____: portion of the brain that contains the primary visual center and is involved in the interpretation of visual data.

4. _____: pathway and processing station between the cerebral motor cortex and the upper brainstem.

5. _____: portion of the brain responsible for perception and balance, as well as interpretation of sounds, tastes, and smells.

6. _____: ability to identify an object by touch.

7. _____: works with the motor cortex of the cerebrum; involved in voluntary movement; processes information from eyes, ears, and touch.

8. _____: a syndrome simulating degenerative disease that is caused by noncommunicating hydrocephalus (dilated ventricles with intracranial pressure within expected ranges).

9. _____: a severe form of child abuse resulting from the violent shaking of infants younger than 1 year of age.

130

10. _____: a clinical syndrome of intracranial hypertension that mimics brain tumors; potential causes include use of certain medications or metabolic, infectious, or hematologic causes.

11. _____: inability to coordinate muscle activity during voluntary movement.

12. _____: stiff neck; associated with meningitis.

13. _____: relays sensory aspects of motor information between the basal ganglia and cerebellum.

14. _____: referring to behavior used to limit pain; for example, limping to reduce weight bearing on an affected leg.

15. _____: an unexpected gait pattern manifested by an excessive lift of the hip and knee and an inability to walk on the heels.

16. _____: part of the brain that maintains temperature control, water metabolism, and neuroendocrine activity.

17. _____: tactual ability to recognize writing on the skin.

18. _____: pathway between the cerebral cortex and spinal cord.

19. _____: a sign assessed as positive when a patient standing with eyes closed is unable to maintain balance.

20. _____: a sign characterized by involuntary flexion of the hips and knees when the neck is flexed.

21. _____: portion of the brain that contains the motor cortex; associated with voluntary skeletal movement.

22. _____: site where the descending corticospinal tracts decussate.

Anatomy Review 1

Identify the structures of the skull and brain labeled on the illustration by writing the correct term in the blank next to the corresponding letter.

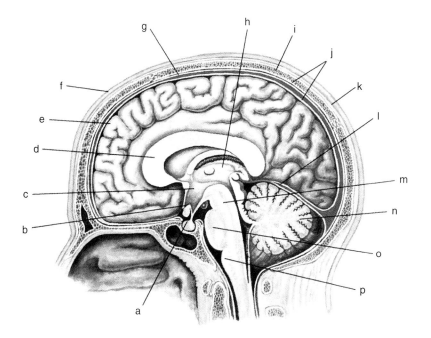

a. _____	Cerebellum
b. _____	Cerebrum
c. _____	Corpus callosum
d. _____	Dura mater (two layers)
e. _____	Galea aponeurotica
f. _____	Hypothalamus
g. _____	Medulla oblongata
h. _____	Midbrain
i. _____	Optic chiasma
j. _____	Pituitary gland
k. _____	Pons
l. _____	Skin
m. _____	Skull
n. _____	Superior sagittal sinus
o. _____	Tentorium cerebelli
p. _____	Thalamus

Anatomy Review 2

Identify the cranial nerves or structures of the skull and brain labeled on the illustration by writing the correct term in the blank next to the corresponding letter.

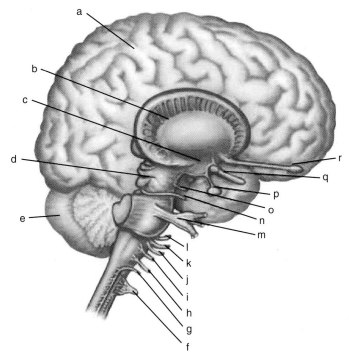

a. _____	Abducens (VI)
b. _____	Acoustic (VIII)
c. _____	Cerebellum
d. _____	Cerebral peduncle
e. _____	Cerebrum
f. _____	Facial (VII)
g. _____	Glossopharyngeal (IX)
h. _____	Hypoglossal (XII)
i. _____	Hypothalamus
j. _____	Oculomotor (III)
k. _____	Olfactory (I)
l. _____	Optic (II)
m. _____	Pituitary gland
n. _____	Spinal accessory (XI)
o. _____	Thalamus
p. _____	Trigeminal (IV)
q. _____	Trochlear (IV)
r. _____	Vagus (X)

Concepts Application 1

Complete the following table by listing the cranial nerve(s) tested by each examination procedure. More than one cranial nerve may be tested by each procedure.

Examination Procedure	Cranial Nerve(s) Tested
Whisper test	
Patient sticks out tongue and moves it toward nose and toward chin	
Taste test with sugar, salt, and lemon	
Visual acuity	
Patient puffs out cheeks and shows teeth	
Patient shrugs shoulders against examiner's hands	
Smell test with coffee, orange, and cloves	
Pupils constrict and dilate in response to light	
Patient clenches teeth (temporal muscles contracted)	

Concepts Application 2

In the table below, write the name of the reflex based on the observed response; then indicate whether this reflex is expected or unexpected based on the age of the infant and/or the nature of the response.

Age of Infant	Observed Response	Name of Reflex	Expected or Unexpected?
2 months	The infant demonstrates a strong grasp of the examiner's finger when it is placed in the infant's palm.		
4 months	When held in an upright position with the soles of the feet touching the surface of a table, the infant flexes the legs upward in a curled position and holds them there.		
6 months	With the child lying supine, turn the head to one side; the arm and leg extend on the side that the head was turned toward.		
8 months	The infant abducts and extends the arms and legs in response to sudden movement of the head and trunk backward. The arms then adduct in an embracing motion followed by relaxation.		

Matching

Match each set of characteristic findings with its corresponding diagnosis.

Characteristic Findings	Diagnosis
_____ 1. Fatigue, bladder dysfunction, sexual dysfunction, sensory changes, muscle weakness	a. Myasthenia gravis
_____ 2. A chronic disorder characterized by recurrent, unprovoked disturbances in consciousness, behavior, sensation, and autonomic functioning secondary to an underlying brain abnormality	b. Generalized seizure disorder
	c. Multiple sclerosis
_____ 3. Fever, chills, headache, and nuchal rigidity	d. Trigeminal neuralgia
_____ 4. Sudden weakness and numbness; confusion; difficulty speaking; loss of balance; paralysis of face, arm, or leg	e. Cerebral vascular accident
	f. Cerebral palsy
_____ 5. An autoimmune disorder of neuromuscular junction involved with muscle activation	g. Meningitis
_____ 6. Progressive bilateral and symmetric distal weakness, diminished reflexes in ascending pattern, difficulty walking	h. Guillain-Barré syndrome
	i. Parkinson disease
_____ 7. Recurrent paroxysmal sharp pain that radiates onto cranial nerve V	
_____ 8. Static and nonprogressive cerebral lesions that cause significant motor delay in a child	
_____ 9. Progressive, degenerative neurologic disorder in older adults	

Case Study

A 64-year-old man is admitted to the hospital with a diagnosis of acute CVA. Listed below are data collected by the examiner during an interview and examination.

INTERVIEW DATA

The patient's wife tells the examiner that her husband was fine until this morning, when he suddenly had a headache, fell to the floor, and could not get up. She adds that when she tried to get her husband to speak, he made only mumbling noises, and she could not understand him.

EXAMINATION DATA

Mental status: Awake, alert man. Unable to talk but able to follow commands. Very distraught over this incident. Patient cries and avoids eye contact with his wife and the examiner.

Neurologic examination: Cranial nerves I, II, III, IV, V, VI, and VII all intact. Patient has asymmetry and unequal movements of his face, with a drooping of the left side of his face. Has asymmetry of shoulder shrug, with deficiency noted on the left side. Patient has left-sided paralysis. Demonstrates expected muscle tone and sensation on right side. Unable to assess balance. Patient unable to get up or move around in bed unassisted at this time.

1. What data deviate from normal findings, suggesting a need for further investigation?

2. What additional questions could the examiner ask to clarify symptoms?

3. What additional physical examination, if any, should the examiner complete?

4. What primary problems does the patient have?

CLINICAL REASONING

1. An ambitious novice examiner uses an unfolded paper clip to test peripheral two-point discrimination. He adjusts the paper clip so that the points are 1 inch apart. With this instrument, he tests the patient's palm, toe, back, upper arm, and upper leg. He notes that the patient fails to discriminate between one and two points in each of these areas. He concludes that the patient has some sort of peripheral sensory deficit. What is incorrect in his methods or conclusion?

2. The computed tomography scan of a patient demonstrates an infarction of the frontal lobe toward the left side. What brain functions occur in the frontal lobe? What type of symptoms would you anticipate this patient to have?

Patient Safety Consideration

1. What must the examiner be ready to do when evaluating a patient with the Romberg test?

2. If a patient has a positive Romberg sign, what should the examiner decide to do in the interest of safety?

CONTENT REVIEW QUESTIONS

Multiple Choice

Circle the best answer for each of the following questions:

1. Which of the following disorders is known to be hereditary?
   a. Peripheral neuropathy
   b. Meningitis
   c. Huntington chorea
   d. Seizure disorder

2. Which cranial nerve is not routinely tested unless a problem is suspected?
   a. I
   b. II
   c. V
   d. XI

3. The patient is able to touch each finger to his thumb in rapid sequence. What does this finding mean? The patient has
   a. intact trochlear and abducens cranial nerves.
   b. appropriate cerebellar function.
   c. an intact spinal accessory nerve.
   d. intact kinesthetic sensation.

4. Which question asked by the examiner may help determine prevention strategies for seizures that a patient has been experiencing?
   a. "Where do your seizures typically begin?"
   b. "How do you feel after the seizure?"
   c. "What goes through your mind during the seizure?"
   d. "Are there any factors or activities that seem to start the seizures?"

5. The examiner asks the patient to close her eyes and then places a vibrating tuning fork on the patient's ankle and asks her to indicate what is felt. What is being assessed?
   a. Peripheral nerve sensory function
   b. Cranial nerve sensory function
   c. Primary sensory function
   d. Level of consciousness

6. A 52-year-old obese man has a history of poorly controlled diabetes, hypertension, and high cholesterol levels. He also smokes. Based on these data, the examiner should recognize that the man has several risk factors for
   a. seizures.
   b. stroke.
   c. multiple sclerosis.
   d. Guillain-Barré syndrome.

7. Which of the following assessment findings should not be surprising to an examiner given the patient's history as described in Question 6?
   a. Inability to discern superficial touch or two-point discrimination on the legs
   b. Reduced muscle tone on left side of the face
   c. Asymmetry of the face when asked to smile and puff out his cheeks
   d. Slow and uncoordinated movement with the finger–nose test

8. The examiner is assessing deep tendon reflex response in a 12-year-old boy. The boy's response is an expected reflex. Which of the following scores should be documented?
   a. 1+
   b. 2+
   c. 3+
   d. 4+

9. An older patient tells the examiner, "I have a hard time figuring out sounds and where they are coming from." This symptom may be
   a. a precursor to a seizure disorder.
   b. an early symptom of Parkinson disease.
   c. an indication of a dysfunction of the temporal lobe.
   d. associated with a problem of the vestibular apparatus.

10. How can an examiner best gain the cooperation of a child when performing a neurologic examination?
    a. Ask a parent to perform the examination while the examiner observes the response.
    b. Ask the mother or father to step out of the room.
    c. Promise the child a toy or treat if he or she does what you ask.
    d. Create a game from various aspects of the neurologic examination.

11. Which of the following infant reflex responses is considered normal?
    a. A 13-month-old baby's toes fan in response to stroking the lateral surface of the infant's sole.
    b. An 8-month-old infant demonstrates a positive Moro reflex when startled.
    c. A 3-month-old infant's fingers fan when the examiner's finger is placed in the infant's hand.
    d. A 2-month-old infant's legs flex up against the body when the infant is held in an upright position, and the dorsal side of the foot is touched to the table.

12. The examiner is conducting an interview with the mother of an infant as part of the neurologic system examination. Which of the following responses made by the mother may indicate a need for further evaluation?
    a. "My baby sometimes falls asleep when I am feeding her."
    b. "My baby seems to jump when there is a loud noise in the room."
    c. "I drank a glass of wine about once a week while I was pregnant."
    d. "I had problems with hypertension the entire time I was pregnant."

13. A patient demonstrates impaired pain sensation. Which additional test is appropriate to further evaluate this finding?
    a. Heat and cold sensation
    b. Ultrasonic perception
    c. Deep tendon reflex
    d. Transillumination of the involved area

14. The examiner squeezes the patient's biceps muscle as part of an examination. Which of the following responses verbalized by the patient is considered normal?
    a. "That makes my arm tingle."
    b. "That makes a burning sensation go up my arm."
    c. "That is uncomfortable."
    d. "My arm is twitching."

15. Which of the following findings is associated with an increased risk for skin breakdown and injury?
    a. Inability to feel pressure applied by a 5.07 monofilament
    b. Inability to identify a familiar object by touch
    c. Inability to identify a letter drawn in the palm of the hand
    d. 3+ deep tendon reflexes

16. A 52-year-old patient with diabetes presents to the office for a routine examination. You have checked protective sensation with 5.07 monofilament, and you noted a loss of sensation. This indicates
    a. peripheral neuropathy.
    b. positive Kernig sign.
    c. positive Brudzinski sign.
    d. posturing.

17. A patient is brought into the emergency department unresponsive following a motor vehicle accident. The patient's arms are fully extended with the forearms pronated. The wrists and fingers are flexed and the jaw is clenched. The neck is extended and the feet are plantar flexed. What does the examiner infer based on these findings?
    a. The patient has a brainstem injury.
    b. The patient has had a seizure.
    c. The patient has damage to the corticospinal tracts.
    d. The patient has a transection of the spinal cord.

18. Which patient response indicates a positive Brudzinski sign?
    a. Involuntary flexion of the hips and knees when the neck is flexed
    b. Headache worsened by hyperextending and then flexing the head
    c. Resistence to dorsiflexing the foot
    d. Pain on adduction of the hip

19. On examination of which patient would an examiner expect to find a positive Kernig sign?
    a. A patient with Parkinson disease
    b. A patient who has had a stroke
    c. A patient with a whiplash injury
    d. A patient with meningitis

20. As a patient walks from the waiting area to the examining room, the examiner notes that the patient's feet are wide apart and his trunk sways as he staggers and lurches side to side. How should the examiner document this observation?
    a. Dystrophic gait
    b. Cerebellar ataxia
    c. Dystonia
    d. Spastic diplegia

24 Putting it All Together

LEARNING OBJECTIVES

After studying Chapter 24 in the textbook and completing this section of the laboratory manual, students should be able to:
1. Discuss the process of completing the history and physical examination.
2. Describe patient reliability and factors that may affect the accuracy of the data collected.
3. Describe the general examination sequence.
4. Identify techniques useful for the evaluation of infants and young children.
5. Discuss functional assessment.

TERMINOLOGY REVIEW

Check your understanding of terminology related to "putting it all together." Using the space provided, write the word or phrase from the list next to the appropriate descriptor.

Activities of daily living (ADLs)
Basic activities of daily living
Cultural barriers
Emotional constraints, apparent and inapparent
Functional assessment
Instrumental activities of daily living
Language barriers
Sensory deprivation

1. _____: patients may speak a language different from yours; translation can be difficult in the best of circumstances; passing messages among three persons often results in changes in meaning that might have serious importance, and confusion may be the result; even using the same language may be a problem if the patient has a limited vocabulary, speaks English as a second language, or cannot read English very well.

2. _____: routine activities that people tend to do every day without needing assistance.

3. _____: a partial or total loss of any of the senses (e.g., vision, hearing, touch, smell) is clearly constraining.

4. _____: patients who are psychotic, delirious, depressed, or in any way seriously emotionally affected may confuse you; emphasize mental status during the history when you suspect this.

5. _____: basic self-care tasks that people normally perform as a routine part of independent living.

6. _____: essential examination of every older adult whether the person is coping well or not coping well in the community environment.

7. _____: housekeeping, grocery shopping, meal preparation, medication compliance, communication skills, and money management.

8. _____: pay attention to the possibility of cultural differences between you and the patient; approach the variety of life experience with candor and interested, compassionate inquiry.

Matching

A 62-year-old man requires a routine physical examination. Listed below are some of the procedures that will be performed during the examination, as well as some of the equipment that will be needed. Match each examination procedure with the type of equipment needed for the procedure. Some equipment will be used more than once; some procedures require more than one answer.

Examination Procedure	Equipment Needed
_____ 1. Red reflex	a. Eye chart (Snellen)
_____ 2. Lung sounds	b. Gloves
_____ 3. Jugular venous pulsations	c. Lubricant
_____ 4. Symmetry of muscle groups	d. Marking pen
_____ 5. Gag reflex	e. Measuring tape
_____ 6. Thyroid	f. Ophthalmoscope
_____ 7. Rectal and prostate examination	g. Otoscope
_____ 8. Tympanic membrane	h. Penlight
_____ 9. Visual acuity	i. Percussion hammer
_____ 10. Rinne and Weber tests	j. Stethoscope
_____ 11. Liver span	k. Tongue blade
_____ 12. Lymph nodes	l. Tuning fork
_____ 13. Heart murmurs	m. No equipment needed
_____ 14. Deep tendon reflex	
_____ 15. Romberg test	
_____ 16. Retinal examination	
_____ 17. Bowel sounds	
_____ 18. Tactile fremitus	

Concepts Application

Complete the following table by identifying the body systems examined in each of the examination areas listed in the left column. Select the appropriate body systems from the list provided below. You will use some systems more than once.

Auditory	Mouth and oropharynx
Breasts and axillae	Musculoskeletal
Cardiovascular	Neurologic
Gastrointestinal	Nose and paranasal
Integumentary	Respiratory
Lymphatic	Visual

Examination Area	Body Systems Examined
Upper extremities	
Anterior chest	
Abdomen	
Head and neck	

CLINICAL REASONING

1. A 61-year-old blind woman presents for a yearly physical examination. What type of modification, if any, should be made to individualize your examination approach or procedures for this individual?

2. A 43-year-old man presents for his 6-month physical examination. He has multiple health problems, including diabetes and coronary artery disease. From the onset of the examination, the patient is overbearing; he begins questioning your techniques and your abilities. He indicates that he is an important person in the community and knows many other people of importance. What things can you do to gain this individual's confidence and decrease his anxiety?

Multiple Choice

Circle the best answer for each of the following questions.

1. When performing a physical examination, you should consider the examination to begin
   a. as soon as you meet the patient.
   b. after the vital signs are taken.
   c. after you explain to the patient everything you are going to do.
   d. after the patient has put on an examination gown.

2. The examiner may decide to omit various aspects of an examination. Which of the following is the best reason for this decision?
   a. The patient is feeling ill.
   b. The patient already knows what is wrong, and a diagnosis can be based on the history.
   c. Certain examination steps will provide data of limited value.
   d. Anxiety is observed by the examiner.

3. In what way can the patient's modesty be maintained while an examination is being conducted? The examiner should
   a. turn his or her back while the patient undresses.
   b. keep the patient covered as much as possible during the examination.
   c. avoid touching the patient during the examination except when absolutely necessary.
   d. not require the patient to disrobe for the examination.

4. Which examination approach is suggested for a 14-month-old baby? The baby should be
   a. completely undressed and lying down on an examination table.
   b. fully clothed and placed on the floor with toys; the examiner should conduct the examination while the child plays.
   c. completely undressed and held by the examiner.
   d. wearing only a diaper and sitting on his or her parent's lap.

5. Which examination technique is not generally included in the examination of a newborn infant?
   a. Percussion of the chest
   b. Palpation of the abdomen
   c. Auscultation of the lungs
   d. Inspection of the mouth and palate

6. Which of the following assists the examiner in determining the gestational age of a newborn infant?
   a. Measurement of the head circumference
   b. Percussion to determine liver size
   c. Inspection of hair distribution of the scalp
   d. Inspection of the sole of the foot

7. A patient complains of a sore throat. Which aspect of the examination could be eliminated?
   a. Vital signs
   b. Palpation of lymph nodes
   c. Deep tendon reflexes
   d. Auscultation of the heart and lungs

8. All of the following can be assessed initially during the general inspection *except*
   a. mobility.
   b. nutritional status.
   c. urinary function.
   d. skin color.

9. What technique will most likely facilitate the examination of a small frightened girl?
   a. Promise the child you won't hurt her.
   b. Tell the child a story in order to distract her.
   c. Use restraints to hold the child but tell her you are playing a game with her.
   d. Tell the child you will give her a toy or treat if she does not cry.

10. Which of the following is generally more relevant to the examination of older adults than to other age groups?
    a. Functional assessment
    b. Physical measurements
    c. Developmental scoring
    d. Vital signs, including peripheral pulse examination

11. For a routine physical examination, all of the following equipment is necessary *except*
    a. a penlight.
    b. a measuring tape.
    c. examination gloves.
    d. a monofilament.

12. Which problem is suggested by assessment findings of irritability, jitteriness, and poor sucking in a newborn?
    a. Placental insufficiency prior to birth
    b. Herpes simplex virus exposure during birth
    c. Neonatal abstinence syndrome
    d. Hypothermia

13. Which is a guideline to be followed when examining a patient?
    a. Sequence the examination in an order that progresses smoothly and conserves patient energy.
    b. Examine from the critical to less critical: follow the ABCs.
    c. Start the examination with the system identified by the chief complaint and progress through related systems.
    d. Assess each system independently, proceeding in a cephalocaudal and proximodistal direction.

14. The Ballard Gestational Age Score is completed within 36 hours of birth to
    a. determine if the menstrual-estimated age is correct.
    b. determine if the newborn is premature.
    c. determine if weight is appropriate for age.
    d. determine if reflexes are developmentally normal.

15. To what does sensitivity refer when used to describe a diagnostic test?
    a. Effectiveness of the test in comparison to similar tests
    b. Effectiveness of the test in clarifying clinical examination findings
    c. Likelihood of obtaining a false positive about an abnormality
    d. Likelihood that the test will detect an abnormality if it exists

Sports Participation Evaluation

<u>LEARNING OBJECTIVES</u>

After studying Chapter 25 in the textbook and completing this section of the laboratory manual, students should be able to:
1. Describe health history and physical examination techniques for the participation examination.
2. Discuss the required components of the preparticipation examination.
3. Describe a 14-step musculoskeletal examination.
4. Review pathologic conditions and determination for sports participation.

<u>TERMINOLOGY REVIEW</u>

Check your understanding of terminology related to the sports participation evaluation. Using the space provided, write the word or phrase from the list next to the appropriate descriptor.

Atlantoaxial instability
Oligomenorrhea
Primary amenorrhea
RED-S
Sports-related concussion

1. _____: no onset of menses by 16 years of age.

2. _____: a syndrome affecting male and female athletes resulting from insufficient caloric intake and/or excessive energy expenditure.

3. _____: a complex pathophysiologic process affecting the brain induced by traumatic biomechanical forces.

4. _____: condition in which the joint is excessively mobile; there may be no neurologic complications at first, but risk exists for subluxation and spinal cord compression.

5. _____: interval between periods greater than 35 days.

For each component of the preparticipation history listed, identify specific questions to be asked/data to be included.

Preparticipation Component	Questions to be Asked/Data to be Included
Medical History	
General Questions	
Heart Health (Self and Family)	
Bone and Joint	
Medical Questions	
Females only	

A 17-year-old adolescent presents for a preparticipation examination for wrestling. On examination, his blood pressure is 126/82 mm Hg. His height is 5 feet, 9 inches (50th percentile for age), and his weight is 65 kg (50th percentile for age). His blood pressure at his last visit 1 year ago was 110/70 mm Hg. He is asymptomatic today.

a. How should his hypertension be classified?

b. What are the next steps in evaluating his elevated blood pressure?

c. Use of what substances would you ask the athlete about?

d. What classification of contact is wrestling?

CONTENT REVIEW QUESTIONS

Multiple Choice

Circle the best answer for each of the following questions:

1. The main purpose in determining the normal neuro-psychologic status in the preparticipation examination is to
   a. clear the individual for all sports participation.
   b. allow you to better judge the return to normal in the event of injury.
   c. judge the ability of the individual to play contact sports.
   d. ensure that subsequent preparticipation examinations can be brief.

2. Which component of the preparticipation examination contributes most to identifying an athlete's risk for injury?
   a. Neurologic evaluation
   b. Musculoskeletal examination
   c. Patient's medical history
   d. General physical examination

3. Which are frequent manifestations of the female athlete triad?
   a. eating disorder, amenorrhea, and osteoporosis.
   b. thyroid dysfunction, eating disorder, and amenorrhea.
   c. stress fractures, thyroid dysfunction, and oligomenorrhea.
   d. eating disorder, thyroid dysfunction, and osteoporosis.

4. In female athletes during teenage years, an overly thin body frame encourages
   a. primary amenorrhea.
   b. thyroid dysfunction.
   c. an eating disorder.
   d. a low estrogen state.

5. A 12-year-old patient with Down syndrome is brought in for a preperformance evaluation in preparation for participation in soccer. On examination, you find increased deep tendon reflexes, a positive Babinski sign, and ankle clonus. Which action should you take?
   a. Initiate a consult with a neurosurgeon experienced with atlantoaxial instability.
   b. Recommend a program of balance and stability exercises with reevaluation before engaging in soccer.
   c. Refer immediately to a neurosurgeon with expertise in atlantoaxial instability.
   d. Request an orthopedic evaluation be obtained, with the report sent to you for follow-up.
   injury.

6. Which of the following is true regarding the preparticipation examination?
   a. The only necessary component is a musculoskeletal examination.
   b. There is nothing legally binding about the provider's recommendation.
   c. Noncontact sports do not require a preparticipation examination.
   d. The only place to perform a preparticipation examination is in a clinic.

7. How often should middle and high school athletes have a comprehensive preparticipation examination (PPE)?
   a. Every year
   b. Following any injury
   c. Varies by sport
   d. Varies by state

8. Sudden cardiac death in athletes is a great concern. Which of the following precludes an athlete from participation in sports?
   a. Hypertension
   b. Carditis
   c. Heart murmur
   d. Dysrhythmia

9. Participation in which sport would be considered to involve the least risk for a 19-year-old patient with atlantoaxial instability?
   a. Soccer
   b. Swimming
   c. Softball
   d. Skiing

10. Which of the following conditions is a reason to deny a patient the ability to play sports?
    a. Previous concussion
    b. Heat-related illness
    c. Fever
    d. Hypertension

11. Harry is a 16-year-old patient who is returning for hypertension that is stage 2. This is defined as
    a. blood pressure greater than the 99th percentile.
    b. blood pressure greater than the 95th percentile.
    c. blood pressure higher than 5 mm Hg.
    d. blood pressure greater than 110/80 mm Hg.

12. Which of the following are classified as limited contact sports?
    a. Ultimate Frisbee and canoeing in white water
    b. Bicycling and racquetball
    c. Badminton and baseball
    d. Lacrosse and diving

Emergency or Life-Threatening Situations

LEARNING OBJECTIVES

After studying Chapter 26 in the textbook and completing this section of the laboratory manual, students should be able to:
1. Compare and contrast primary and secondary assessment.
2. Describe findings considered significant in the secondary assessment.
3. Describe how pediatric emergency assessment differs from adult emergency assessment.
4. Identify pediatric findings considered to be of concern or ominous.
5. Discuss the impact of advance directives on providing immediate care.

TERMINOLOGY REVIEW

Check your understanding of terminology related to assessment in emergency and life-threatening situations. Using the space provided, write the word or phrase from the list next to the appropriate descriptor.

ABCs
Advance directive
Blunt trauma
Durable power of attorney
Hypoxemia
Increased intracranial pressure
Penetrating trauma
Primary assessment

Pulmonary embolism
Secondary assessment
Shock state
Status asthmaticus
Status epilepticus
Upper airway obstruction
Ventilatory failure

1. _____: injury that penetrates the patient's skin.

2. _____: severely reduced blood oxygen levels in major organs, resulting from respiratory distress, poor tissue perfusion, or ventilatory failure.

3. _____: compromise of the airway space resulting in impaired respiratory exchange.

4. _____: abnormality of the circulatory system that results in inadequate organ perfusion and tissue oxygenation; common causes include hemorrhage associated with injury.

5. _____: compromised exhalation of carbon dioxide caused by alveolar hypoventilation.

6. _____: more detailed head-to-toe examination to identify problems.

7. _____: a provision for another person to make healthcare decisions in the event that the patient's cognition is lost.

8. _____: injury that does not penetrate the skin.

9. _____: acute severe asthma exacerbation that does not respond to usual treatment.

10. _____: rapid evaluation of the patient's physiologic status (the ABCs).

11. _____: a condition in which an increase in the volume of brain tissue, blood, or cerebrospinal fluid within the closed space of the skull results in elevated pressure.

12. _____: migration of a blood clot from the deep veins of the legs or pelvis to the lung vasculature.

13. _____: a formal statement of desired medical care in the event of catastrophic injury or illness.

14. _____: a prolonged seizure (or a series of seizures) that occurs without recovery of consciousness.

15. _____: airway, breathing, circulation.

APPLICATION TO CLINICAL PRACTICE

Concepts Application

Indicate whether the action described would be part of a primary or secondary assessment in a patient with a life-threatening condition.

1. _____ Removing clothing from a patient with an abdominal gunshot wound

2. _____ Performing a Glasgow Coma Scale assessment

3. _____ Taking a history of injury

4. _____ Stabilizing the cervical spine

5. _____ Auscultating the heart

6. _____ Taking vital signs

7. _____ Managing a large, pulsating, bleeding wound

8. _____ Assessing for presence of breathing

9. _____ Assessing the abdomen for internal bleeding

10. _____ Assessing carotid or femoral pulse

Case Study

Mark O'Neil is a 19-year-old man rushed to the emergency department by his roommate.

PRIMARY ASSESSMENT

Upon arrival, Mark is extremely anxious and has profound dyspnea. He states, "Please help me. I can't breathe enough air—something is wrong with me! My chest hurts all over, and I can't breathe!" The examiner notes a large, muscular, healthy-appearing man in acute respiratory distress. Nasal flaring is noted with cyanosis around the lips. Overall impression is that of hypoxia.

1. Based on this information, list your primary assessment findings:
   A:

B:

C:

2. What type of treatment should be initiated immediately during the primary assessment?

3. What is the first thing that should be assessed at the onset of the secondary assessment?

<u>SECONDARY ASSESSMENT: SUBJECTIVE DATA</u>

Mark's roommate tells you that Mark is very athletic and very healthy. "He plays college football and had surgery on his knee 2 weeks ago because of an injury this past season. This evening he was fine—we were watching TV. Then when he got up to go into the kitchen, he called for help and told me to get him to the hospital now! All that happened about 20 minutes ago." The roommate says that Mark does not use any drugs. He adds, "He drinks beer and stuff, but nothing tonight."

<u>SECONDARY ASSESSMENT: OBJECTIVE DATA</u>

Vital signs: Pulse 142. Respiratory rate 40. Blood pressure 138/84. Temperature 99.1°F.

Skin color: Generally pale with cyanosis around lips and in nail beds.

Head/neck: Pupils reactive to light. Oral cavity WNL.

Chest: Breath sounds auscultated in all lung fields. Has productive cough with bloody sputum. Heart sounds WNL.

Abdomen: Bowel sounds present. No pain; soft, nondistended.

Extremities: Pulses palpable in all extremities; no swelling.

Neurologic: Awake but not following all commands; extremely anxious.

Arterial blood gas: pH 7.31; O_2 63; PCO_2 69 (respiratory acidosis).

4. What data deviate from normal?

5. What additional secondary assessment would you plan to conduct?

6. Based on the information presented, what problems do you think this patient might be experiencing?

Completion

Complete the following two mnemonics, which are useful in emergency situations. Fill in the meaning of each letter in the mnemonic in the space provided.

1. Initial assessment of a patient's level of responsiveness

   A _____

   V _____

   P _____

   U _____

2. Abbreviated Patient History Information

   A _____

   M _____

   P _____

   L _____

   E _____

CLINICAL REASONING

1. Mrs. Martin and her 3-year-old daughter, Amanda, are brought to the hospital for emergency care after being burned in a house fire.
   a. In addition to the burns, what types of problems should the examiner rule out on both of these patients?

   b. What anatomic differences between Amanda and her mother will affect how they are examined?

CONTENT REVIEW QUESTIONS

Multiple Choice

Circle the best answer for each of the following questions:

1. Approximately how long should an examiner take to conduct a primary assessment of a stable patient?
   a. 30 seconds
   b. 60 seconds
   c. 2 minutes
   d. 5 minutes

2. After the initial primary assessment is conducted, how often should it be repeated?
   a. Every 30 seconds
   b. Every 2 minutes
   c. Every 5 minutes
   d. Every time the patient's condition changes

3. Which finding is consistent with abdominal hemorrhage?
   a. Increased bowel sounds
   b. Distention and pain
   c. Hyperresonance with percussion
   d. Auscultation of mesentery artery

4. Which of the following findings suggests a serious problem in a 3-year-old child who has fallen from a tree?
   a. Respiratory rate of 38 breaths/min
   b. Pulse rate of 150 beats/min
   c. Lethargy
   d. Crying

5. Mike complains of severe rib pain. His coworkers state that he was hurt on the job when a large pipe struck him across the chest. Given this history, which type of problem should be considered during the secondary assessment?
   a. Flail chest
   b. Rebound tenderness
   c. Pulmonary embolus
   d. Pupillary constriction

6. A patient who was involved in a motor vehicle accident presents with a suspected neck injury. Which of the following actions by the examiner is clearly *not* appropriate?
   a. Assessing peripheral pulses
   b. Providing airway support
   c. Logrolling the patient to assess his back
   d. Hyperextending the neck to establish an airway

7. With which of the following clinical problems would crepitation be an expected finding?
   a. Myocardial infarction
   b. Cardiovascular accident
   c. Blunt abdominal trauma
   d. Pneumothorax

8. During the primary assessment, the examiner asks the patient, "Can you tell me who you are?" This question assesses
   a. airway and orientation.
   b. exposure and circulation.
   c. breathing and circulation.
   d. disability and exposure.

9. Which of the following findings suggests poor peripheral perfusion?
   a. Rapid heart rate
   b. Dorsalis pedis pulse with 3 + amplitude
   c. Capillary refill time longer than 2 seconds
   d. Palpable ulnar pulse

10. A child is struck by a car while riding his bike. Upon arrival at the hospital, the child is not breathing. Which of the following best describes the appropriate actions of an examiner?
    a. Conduct a primary and secondary assessment before deciding what care to provide.
    b. Conduct a primary assessment; before starting a secondary assessment, support breathing.
    c. Stop the primary assessment as soon as the apnea is recognized in order to perform interventions to stabilize the breathing.
    d. Appropriate action depends on the degree of cyanosis observed by the examiner.

11. An examiner suspects that a patient has a cervical spine injury. The examiner can rule out this possibility by
    a. examining peripheral motor function and sensation.
    b. assessing level of consciousness.
    c. assessing for pain and deformity.
    d. acquiring radiographic films of all cervical vertebrae.

12. During primary assessment, the examiner notes dampness inside a trauma victim's dark-colored coat. Which of the following possible causes for the dampness would be most important for the examiner to determine?
    a. Severe sweating
    b. Urine
    c. IV fluids
    d. Blood

13. A patient presents with a complaint of sudden flashes of light in the field of vision. What other symptom commonly accompanies this primary symptom?
    a. Severe nausea and vomiting
    b. Partial loss of vision
    c. Severe pain to the eye
    d. Intense dizziness

14. A man is shot and critically wounded during a domestic dispute. From a legal standpoint, the healthcare providers must
    a. obtain written consent from the patient before providing care.
    b. call the police before providing care.
    c. save all items obtained from the patient for law enforcement personnel.
    d. determine whether the man has advance directives before providing care.

15. Which patient history information is an essential part of the primary assessment?
    a. Chief concern
    b. Drug allergies
    c. Present medical history
    d. Family history

Student Performance Checklists

Health History Guide	Assessed Appropriately by Student?		Comments
	Yes	No	
I. Beginning data			
A. Date and time			
B. Source of data (patient, family member, etc.)			
C. Name and role of interviewer			
II. Patient's identifying information and biographic data (cultural background, family structure, education, and economic and environmental data may be listed in the personal and social history section.)			
A. Name			
B. Sex assigned at birth			
C. Sexual orientation			
D. Gender identity			
E. Age			
D. Birth date and place			
E. Race and culture			
F. Religion			
G. Education			
H. Marital status			
I. Occupation			
J. Address and phone number			
K. Socioeconomic data (income, members of household, means of transportation, etc.)			
L. Other (source of referral, previous healthcare provider)			
III. Present illness			
A. Chief concern (CC)			
B. Symptoms (nature, course, location, and pattern of problem)			
1. Date and timing (gradual or sudden onset, duration, frequency)			
2. Character, quality, quantity, and location (generalized or radiating pain)			
3. Associated events (setting)			

Continued

153

Health History Guide	Assessed Appropriately by Student?		Comments
	Yes	No	
4. Treatments (remissions)			
5. Effect on other systems (appetite)			
6. Influence on usual activities (sleep)			
7. Other (coping ability)			
IV. Past Medical history			
A. Overall health before the presenting problem			
B. Previous hospitalizations and illnesses/dates			
1. Surgeries/dates			
2. Serious injuries and disabilities/dates			
3. Major childhood illnesses/dates			
4. Major adult illnesses/dates			
5. Other pertinent data			
C. Previous healthcare			
1. Recent health examination (physical, Pap smear, x-rays, TB test, dental, vision, hearing)			
2. Immunizations (polio, diphtheria, tetanus, hepatitis A, hepatitis B, influenza, mumps, rubella, pertussis, Pneumovax, measles, varicella, herpes zoster vaccine, human papilloma virus)			
3. Skin tests (BCG/PPD)			
4. Other (obstetric care, screening tests, laboratory work)			
D. Current health/risk factors			
1. Exercise (how often, duration)			
2. Smoking (how much per day)			
3. Alcohol (how often, amount, type)			
4. Nutrition (caffeine, salt intake, amount)			
5. Sleep pattern (number of hours/night)			
6. Other (work stress, anxiety)			
E. Medication data			
1. OTC drugs (including vitamins)			
2. Prescriptions (dosage, schedule, including birth control pills)			
3. Allergies (transfusions, seasonal or environmental, food, dyes, medications)			
4. Other (illegal drug use)			
V. Family history			
A. Status of family members			
1. Family tree (narrative, pedigree)			

Health History Guide	Assessed Appropriately by Student?		Comments
	Yes	No	
2. Major health conditions (heart disease, high blood pressure, cancer, tuberculosis, stroke, sickle cell disease, cystic fibrosis, epilepsy, diabetes, gout, kidney disease, thyroid disease, asthma or other allergic condition, forms of arthritis, blood diseases, sexually transmitted infections, familial hearing, and visual or other sensory problems)			
3. Genetic disorders (sickle cell disease)			
VI. Personal and social history			
If not addressed previously or if more information is needed, describe cultural background, family structure, stress factors, educational data, economic status, and environmental data (home, school, work, "typical day").			
VII. Review of physiologic systems			
A. General, overall trends			
1. Vital signs (temperature, pulse [apical and radial], blood pressure, and respirations)			
2. Previous measurements (height and weight; head, chest, limb circumferences)			
3. Usual health status (fatigue or fever patterns)			
4. Other (recent change in usual condition)			
B. Nutritional status			
1. Usual diet (hour-by-hour diary)			
2. Appetite trends			
3. Food choices (preference foods)			
C. Skin, hair, and nails			
1. Usual condition of skin, hair, and nails			
2. Previous diseases or problems (rash or eruption, itching, pigmentation or texture change, excessive sweating, abnormal nail or hair growth)			
3. New or recurrent conditions			
D. Lymphatic system			
1. Usual condition of lymphatic system (i.e., presence of lymphedema)			
2. Previous lumps or nodules (neck or groin area associated with an infection)			
3. Other (*lymph node* enlargement, tenderness, suppuration)			
E. Head and neck			
1. Usual condition of head and neck			
2. Previous diseases or problems (headaches, dizziness, syncope, trauma)			

Continued

Chapter **Student Performance Checklists**

Health History Guide	Assessed Appropriately by Student?		Comments
	Yes	No	
3. New or recurrent conditions			
F. Eyes			
1. Usual condition of eyes, any discharge			
2. Previous diseases, problems (glaucoma or trauma)			
3. New or recurrent conditions			
G. Ears, nose, and throat			
1. Usual condition of ears, nose, and throat			
2. Previous diseases, problems (tinnitus, vertigo, infections, or surgeries)			
3. New or recurrent conditions (nasal polyps, hearing loss)			
4. Other (associated allergies, condition of mouth and teeth)			
H. Chest and lungs			
1. Usual condition of respiratory system			
2. Previous disease or problems (cough, shortness of breath, infections)			
3. New or recurrent conditions (pain related to respiration)			
4. Other (last chest X-ray)			
I. Heart and blood vessels			
1. Usual condition of cardiovascular system			
2. Previous diseases and problems (chest pain or distress, palpitations, dyspnea, edema, hypertension, previous myocardial infarction)			
3. New or recurrent conditions (chest pain, orthopnea)			
4. Other (last ECG)			
J. Breasts			
1. Usual condition of breasts			
2. Previous diseases, problems (pain, tenderness, discharge, lumps, galactorrhea)			
3. New or recurrent conditions (tenderness, new lump or nodule)			
4. Other (last mammogram/date, breast self-awareness, clinical breast examination)			
K. Gastrointestinal			
1. Usual condition of alimentary tract (appetite, digestion)			

Health History Guide	Assessed Appropriately by Student?		Comments
	Yes	No	
2. Previous diseases or problems (ulcers, dysphagia, heartburn, nausea, vomiting, hematemesis, flatulence, constipation, diarrhea, hemorrhoids, jaundice, gallstones, polyps, tumor)			
3. New or recurrent conditions (abdominal pain, change in stool color or contents)			
4. Other (previous diagnostic imaging)			
L. Genitourinary (female)			
1. Usual condition of genitourinary system (including menstruation)			
2. Previous diseases or problems (lesions, sexually transmitted infections, pain, discharges)			
3. New or recurrent conditions (irregular menses)			
4. Other (sexual and childbearing history)			
M. Genitourinary (male)			
1. Usual condition of genitalia (erections and ejaculation data)			
2. Previous diseases or problems (infertility)			
N. Endocrine			
1. Usual condition of endocrine system			
2. Previous diseases or problems (diabetes)			
3. New or recurrent conditions (thyroid enlargement or tenderness, heat or cold intolerance, unexplained weight change, polydipsia, polyuria, changes in facial or body hair, skin striae)			
4. Other (increased hat and glove size)			
O. Musculoskeletal system			
1. Usual condition of musculoskeletal system (gait)			
2. Previous diseases or problems (joint stiffness, restriction of motion)			
3. New or recurrent conditions (pain, swelling, redness, heat)			
4. Other (deformities; limitations; use of devices, e.g., canes, walkers)			
P. Neurologic system			
1. Usual condition of central nervous system			
2. Previous diseases or problems (seizures, tremors, tingling sensations)			

Continued

Chapter **Student Performance Checklists**

Health History Guide	Assessed Appropriately by Student?		Comments
	Yes	No	
3. New or recurrent conditions (loss of memory, weakness, or paralysis)			
4. Other (previous motor, sensory, and cognitive test results)			
Q. Physiologic symptoms			
1. Usual mental and psychological abilities			
2. Previous diseases or problems			
3. New or recurrent conditions			
4. Other (symptoms of Alzheimer disease)			
R. Cross-system data			
1. Data that depict endocrine changes (symptoms that may suggest thyroid disease or diabetes)			

NOTE: This outline can be used as a guide for recording findings related to a patient's age and condition.
Add data that are pertinent to the patient and omit the parts of the outline that are not applicable.

Pain	Assessed Appropriately by Student?		Comments
	Yes	No	
I. Ask the patient if he or she is currently in any pain.			
II. Assess present problem for the following:			
A. Fever			
1. Onset			
2. Associated symptoms			
3. Medications used			
B. Pain			
1. Onset			
2. Quality			
3. Intensity			
4. Location			
5. Associated symptoms			
6. What the patient thinks is causing the pain			
7. Effect of pain on daily activities			
8. Effect of pain on psyche			
9. Pain control measures used			
10. Medications used			
III. Use a pain scale to elicit consistent information on the patient's pain level.			
IV. Differentiate between acute and chronic pain.			
V. Assess behavior patterns for pain.			
VI. Assess for classic pain patterns.			

General Assessment	Assessed Appropriately by Student?		Comments
	Yes	No	
I. Temperature			
A. Oral			
B. Rectal			
C. Axillary			
D. Tympanic			
E. Forehead			
II. Radial pulse (rate, rhythm, quality)			
III. Respiratory rate			
IV. Blood pressure (sitting)			
A. Right arm			
B. Left arm			
V. Height			
VI. Weight			
If applicable: dry weight if on dialysis			

CHAPTER 07

Adult Examination Checklist

Mark data, when appropriate, to indicate the following:
$\times$ If normal, * if abnormal, O if absent.

Subjective Data	Objective Data

__Alertness
__Emotional status
__Orientation
   __Time
   __Place
   __Person
__Analogies (similarities)
__Abstract reasoning (fable, proverb)
__Arithmetic calculations
__Writing ability
__Motor skills
__Memory
   __Immediate
   __Recent
   __Remote
__Attention span (short commands)
__Judgment/decision making (hypothetical situation)
__Voice
   __Quality
   __Pace
   __Loudness
__Articulation
__Comprehension
__Coherence (perceptions clearly conveyed)
__Mood and feelings
__Thought processes (logical)
__Perceptual distortions (hallucinations)
	Observation
	__Alertness
	__Grooming
	__Body language
	__Emotional status
	__Attention span
	__Coherence
	__Voice
	   __Quality
	   __Pace
	   __Loudness
	__Articulation
	__Comprehension
	__Mood and feelings
	__Thought processes
	__Perceptual distortions
	Testing
	__Orientation
	   __Time
	   __Place
	   __Person
	__Analogies
	__Abstract reasoning
	__Arithmetic calculations
	__Writing ability
	__Motor skills
	__Memory
	   __Immediate
	   __Recent
	   __Remote
	__Attention span

Detail those data marked as abnormal:

	Assessed Appropriately by Student?		Comments
	Yes	No	
I. Inspection and palpation of the skin			
A. Color			
B. Uniformity			
C. Thickness			
D. Symmetry			
E. Hygiene			
F. Lesions			
1. Primary			
2. Secondary			
3. Size			
4. Shape			
5. Color			
6. Texture			
7. Elevation or depression			
8. Attachment at base			
9. Exudates			
10. Configuration			
11. Location and distribution			
G. Odors			
H. Moisture			
I. Temperature			
J. Texture			
K. Turgor			
L. Mobility			
II. Inspection and palpation of the hair			
A. Color			
B. Distribution			
C. Quantity			
D. Texture			
III. Inspection and palpation of the nails			
A. Pigmentation, length, symmetry, and ridging or irregularities (redness, swelling, pain, exudate, warts, cysts, or tumors)			
B. Measure nail base angle			
C. Texture, firmness, thickness, uniformity, and adherence to nail bed			

165

	Assessed Appropriately by Student?		Comments
	Yes	No	
I. Inspection and palpation of superficial lymph nodes			
A. Size			
B. Consistency (hard, firm, soft, resilient, spongy, cystic)			
C. Pain, especially on touch or on rebound			
D. Location			
E. Character (smooth, nodular, regular)			
F. Symmetry between sides			
G. Mobility and tenderness			
H. Temperature			
I. Pulsatile nature			
J. Vascularity: degree of redness			
II. Inspection of visible nodes			
A. Visibility and position			
B. Enlargement			
C. Lymphedema			
D. Lymphangitis or red streaks			
E. Skin lesions			
III. Lymph nodes of head and neck			
IV. Lymph nodes of the axillary area			
V. Lymph nodes of the upper/lower extremities			

	Assessed Appropriately by Student?		Comments
	Yes	No	
I. Inspection and palpation of the head and scalp			
A. Head position and tremor			
B. Skull and scalp symmetry, shape, lesions, and trauma; skull size			
C. Facial symmetry, shape, unusual features, pigmentation, and tics			
D. Frontal and maxillary sinuses and mastoid process for palpation without tenderness			
E. Scalp symmetry, tenderness (particularly over areas of frontal and maxillary sinuses), movement; hair texture, color, and distribution			
F. Temporal arteries			
G. Salivary glands			
II. Inspection and palpation of the neck			
A. Neck symmetry, fullness, and ROM (masses, webbing, and skinfolds)			
B. Trachea position or tugging (protrusions, asymmetry)			
C. Movement of hyoid bone and cartilages with swallowing			
D. Lymph nodes			
E. Paravertebral musculature and spinous processes			
F. Thyroid size, shape, and configuration (consistency, nodules, enlargement, tenderness)			
G. Carotid artery condition (distention or asymmetry)			
H. Anterior triangle and posterior triangle			
III. Auscultation of head and neck areas			
A. Temporal artery for bruits			
B. Over the eyes for bruits			
C. Thyroid for bruits			
IV. Palpation of the temporomandibular joint for crepitus			

	Assessed Appropriately by Student?		Comments
	Yes	No	
I. Vision testing			
A. Visual acuity (Snellen chart, E chart, animal and object test, Rosenbaum near-vision chart)			
B. Visual fields (confrontation test)			
II. Inspection and palpation of the eyes			
A. Eyebrows for size, hair texture, and extension to temporal canthus			
B. Orbital area (edema, redundant tissues, or lesions)			
C. Eyelids (ability to open and close, eyelash position, ptosis, fasciculation, tremors, flakiness, redness, swelling); palpate for nodules			
D. Conjunctivae and sclerae: color and condition (discharge, pterygium, lacrimal gland punctum, foreign bodies)			
E. External eyes: corneal clarity, sensitivity, arcus; color of irides; pupillary size and shape, response to light and accommodation, nystagmus			
F. Lacrimal gland condition			
G. Extraocular muscles (corneal light reflex, cover–uncover test, six cardinal fields of gaze)			
III. Ophthalmoscopic inspection (hold the ophthalmoscope in the hand that corresponds to the examining eye)			
A. Lens clarity			
B. Red reflex			
C. Retinal color, lesions			
D. Blood vessel characteristics			
E. Disc characteristics			
F. Macula characteristics (ask the patient to look directly at the light)			
G. Depth of anterior chamber			

	Assessed Appropriately by Student?		Comments
	Yes	No	
I. Inspection, palpation, and testing of the ears			
A. Auricles and mastoid area: size, shape, symmetry, landmarks, color, position, deformities or lesions; palpate noting tenderness, swelling, or nodules			
B. Auditory canal (cerumen, discharge, foreign bodies, lesions, color)			
C. Tympanic membrane: landmarks, color, contour, perforations, and mobility			
D. Assess hearing			
1. Response to questions during history			
2. Weber test: tuning fork midline of skull			
3. Rinne test: tuning fork over mastoid process and then placed in front of the ear			
4. Whisper or watch test			
II. Inspection, palpation, and testing of nose			
A. External nose (size, shape, color); palpate for tenderness, bone or cartilage displacement, and masses			
B. Patency of nares			
C. Nasal mucosa and septum (color alignment, discharge, turbinates, perforation)			
D. Frontal and maxillary sinuses (tenderness, swelling)			
III. Inspection and palpation of the mouth and throat			
A. Internal and external lips: color, symmetry, edema			
B. Teeth (occlusion, caries, loose or missing teeth, surface abnormalities)			
C. Gingivae (color, lesions, tenderness)			
D. Tongue and buccal mucosa (color, symmetry, swelling, ulcerations)			
E. Assess function of cranial nerve XII			
F. Uvula and palate			
G. Tonsils (if present) and posterior wall of pharynx			
H. Elicit gag reflex			

	Assessed Appropriately by Student?		Comments
	Yes	No	
I. Inspection and palpation of the chest (patient sitting with arms across chest for lateral and posterior assessment; patient supine with arms slightly away from chest for anterior assessment)			
A. Anatomic landmarks: trachea, suprasternal notch, angle of Louis, costal angle, C7, T1			
B. Shape, size, symmetry, AP diameter, color of front and back, superficial venous patterns, prominence of ribs			
C. Respiratory rate, rhythm			
D. Chest movement for symmetry and use of accessory muscles			
E. Audible sounds (stridor, wheezes)			
F. Thoracic expansion			
G. Crepitus			
H. Tactile fremitus "99"			
II. Percussion, auscultation, and measurement of the chest			
A. Measurement of diaphragmatic excursion			
B. Intensity, pitch, duration, and quality of percussion tones			
C. Unexpected breath sounds (crackles, rhonchi, wheezes, friction rubs)			
D. Vocal resonance			

	Assessed Appropriately by Student?		Comments
	Yes	No	
I. Inspection and palpation of the heart (patient sitting, leaning forward, and supine)			
A. Precordium (apical impulse, pulsations, heaves, lifts, thrills)			
B. Percuss to estimate heart size			
II. Auscultation of the heart (also in left lateral recumbent position)			
A. Rate, rhythm, splitting			
B. Sounds: S_1, S_2, S_3, and S_4; extra heart sounds (snaps, clicks, friction rubs, or murmurs)			
C. Characteristics of murmurs (timing and duration, pitch, intensity, pattern, quality, location, radiation, variation with respiratory phase)			

	Assessed Appropriately by Student?		Comments
	Yes	No	
I. Inspection, palpation, and auscultation of arteries and veins			
A. Palpate pulses in distal extremities, comparing bilaterally for rate, rhythm, contour, and amplitude.			
B. Auscultate the carotid, abdominal aorta, renal, iliac, and femoral arteries for bruits.			
C. Jugular pulsations and distention, pulse waves (jugular vs. carotid), and pressure			
D. Inspect peripheral veins and arteries for sufficiency (color, skin texture, and nail changes, hair, muscular atrophy, edema, varicosities).			
E. Palpate the extremities for warmth, pulse quality, tenderness, pitting edema.			

	Assessed Appropriately by Student?		Comments
	Yes	No	
I. Inspection and palpation of female breast (with patient seated)			
A. Size, contour, and symmetry			
B. Skin color, texture (dimpling, retractions, supernumerary nipples, venous patterns, lesions or sores)			
C. Nipple and areolae characteristics (shape, symmetry, color, smoothness, size, inversion, eversion, retraction)			
D. Reinspect breasts with the patient in the following positions:			
1. Arms extended over head or flexed behind the neck			
2. Hands pressed on hips with shoulder rolled forward			
3. Seated and leaning over			
4. In recumbent position			
E. Perform a chest wall sweep.			
F. Perform bimanual digital palpation.			
G. Axillary lymph nodes (down the arm to the elbow, and in the axillary, supraclavicular, and infraclavicular areas)			
H. Palpate breast tissue with patient supine (light, medium, and deep pressure).			
I. I. Depress the nipple into the well behind the areola.			
II. Inspection and palpation of male breasts (with patient sitting with arms hanging freely at the sides)			
A. Breast characteristics (shape, symmetry, color, smoothness, size; nipple inversion, eversion, retraction)			
B. Palpate breasts and over areolae for lumps or nodules.			
C. Axillary lymph nodes (down the arm to the elbow, and in the axillary, supraclavicular, and infraclavicular areas)			

Chapter **Student Performance Checklists**

	Assessed Appropriately by Student?		Comments
	Yes	No	
I. Inspection of the abdomen (patient supine, pillow under head, arms at sides)			
A. Skin characteristics, venous return patterns, symmetry, surface motion			
B. Abdominal muscles (as patient raises head) for masses, hernia, or separation			
II. Auscultation of all quadrants			
A. Bowel sounds and frequency			
B. Arteries (bruits)			
III. Percussion of all quadrants			
A. Tone			
B. Estimation of liver size			
C. Splenic dullness			
D. Gastric air bubble			
IV. Light palpation of all quadrants for muscle resistance, tenderness, masses			
V. Deep palpation of all quadrants			
A. Umbilicus and umbilical ring (bulges, masses)			
B. Liver border			
C. Gallbladder			
D. Spleen			
E. Kidneys			
F. Aortic pulsations			
G. Other masses			
VI. With patient seated, percuss the costovertebral angles for kidney tenderness			

	Assessed Appropriately by Student?		Comments
	Yes	No	
I. Inspection and palpation of the female genitalia (patient in lithotomy position)			
A. Pubic hair characteristics and distribution			
B. Labia: color, symmetry, discharge, and characteristics (swelling, inflammation, irritation)			
C. Urethral meatus and vaginal opening (discharge, lesions, polyps, fistulas)			
D. Milk the Skene glands.			
E. Palpate the Bartholin glands.			
F. Perineum: smoothness, tenderness, lesions, inflammation, and fistulas			
G. Inspect for bulging and urinary incontinence as the patient bears down.			
H. Inspect perineal area and anus for skin characteristics, lesions, fissures, excoriation, and inflammation.			
II. Speculum examination			
A. Cervix characteristics (color, position, size, surface characteristics, discharge, size and shape of os)			
B. Collect necessary specimens.			
C. Vaginal characteristics (color, surface characteristics, secretions)			
III. Bimanual examination			
A. Palpate the vaginal walls for smoothness, tenderness, lesions.			
B. Palpate the cervix for size, shape, length, position, mobility.			
C. Palpate the uterus for location, position, size, shape, contour, mobility, tenderness.			
D. Palpate the ovaries for size, shape, consistency, tenderness.			
E. Palpate adnexal areas for masses and tenderness.			
IV. Rectovaginal examination			
A. Assess sphincter tone.			
B. Palpate the rectovaginal septum for thickness, tone, nodules.			
C. Palpate the posterior aspect of the uterus.			
D. Palpate the anterior and posterior rectal wall for masses, polyps, nodules, strictures, other irregularities, tenderness.			
E. Note characteristics of feces when the gloved finger is removed.			

	Assessed Appropriately by Student?		Comments
	Yes	No	
I. Inspection and palpation of male genitalia			
A. Pubic hair characteristics and distribution			
B. Retract the foreskin if patient is uncircumcised.			
C. Glans of the penis (color, smegma); urethral meatus for discharge			
D. Palpate penis for tenderness, induration.			
E. Strip the urethra for discharge.			
F. Scrotum and ventral surface of penis for color, texture, asymmetry, lesions, unusual thickening, and presence of hernia.			
G. Palpate inguinal canal for hernia (direct or indirect).			
H. Palpate testes, epididymides, and vasa deferentia for consistency, size, tenderness, bleeding, masses, lumpiness, or nodules.			
I. Transilluminate any masses in the scrotum.			
J. Palpate for inguinal lymph nodes.			
K. Elicit the cremasteric reflex bilaterally.			

	Assessed Appropriately by Student?		Comments
	Yes	No	
I. Inspection and palpation of the anus, rectum, and prostate			
A. Sacrococcygeal and perianal areas for skin characteristics, lesions, inflammation, dimpling, and excoriation			
B. Anal characteristics (hemorrhoids, polyps, fissures, lesions, fistulas, skin tags, prolapse)			
C. Insert finger and assess sphincter tone.			
D. Muscular ring for smoothness, evenness of pressure against examining finger			
E. Lateral, posterior, and anterior rectal walls for nodules, masses, polyps, tenderness, or irregularities			
F. In men, palpate the posterior surface of the prostate gland through the anterior rectal wall for size, contour, consistency, and mobility.			
G. In women, palpate the cervix and uterus through the anterior rectal wall for size, shape, position, smoothness, and mobility.			
H. Have the patient bear down and palpate deeper for tenderness or nodules.			
I. Withdraw the finger and examine fecal material for color, consistency, blood, or pus. Occult blood by chemical test if indicated.			

	Assessed Appropriately by Student?		Comments
	Yes	No	
I. Inspection and palpation of the musculoskeletal system			
A. Skeleton and extremities: compare sides for alignment, contour and symmetry, size, gross deformity.			
B. Skin and subcutaneous tissues over muscles and joints for color, number of skinfolds, swelling, masses			
C. Inspect muscles and compare sides for size, symmetry, fasciculations, or spasms.			
D. Palpate all bones, joints, and surrounding muscles for muscle tone, heat, tenderness, swelling, and crepitus.			
E. Test each major joint for active and passive range of motion and compare sides			
F. Test major muscle groups for strength and compare sides			
G. Hands and wrists			
1. Dorsum and palm of hands for contour, position, shape, number, and completeness of digits			
2. Palpate each joint in the hand and wrist			
3. Test range of motion: metacarpophalangeal flexion and hyperextension; thumb opposition; forming a fist; finger adduction and abduction; wrist extension, hyperextension and flexion; radial and ulnar motion			
H. Elbows			
1. Inspect the elbows in flexed and extended position for contour and carrying angle.			
2. Palpate the extensor surface of the ulna, olecranon process, and the medial and lateral epicondyles of the humerus.			
3. Test range of motion: flexion, extension, pronation, and supination			
I. Shoulders			
1. Shoulders and shoulder girdle for contour			
2. Palpate the joint spaces and bones of the shoulders.			
3. Test range of motion: shrugging, forward flexion and hyperextension, abduction and adduction, internal and external rotation.			
4. Test muscle strength: shrugging, abduction with forward flexion, medial rotation, lateral rotation.			
J. Temporomandibular joint			
1. Palpate the joint space for clicking, popping, and pain.			

Continued

191

	Assessed Appropriately by Student?		Comments
	Yes	No	
2. Test range of motion: opening and closing mouth, moving jaw laterally to each side, protruding and retracting jaw.			
3. Test strength of temporalis muscles.			
K. Cervical spine			
1. Neck for alignment, symmetry of skinfolds and muscles			
2. Test range of motion: forward flexion, hyperextension, lateral bending, and rotation			
3. Test strength of sternocleidomastoid and trapezius muscles			
L. Thoracic and lumbar spine			
1. Spine for alignment			
2. Palpate the spinal processes and paravertebral muscles			
3. Percuss for spinal tenderness			
4. Test range of motion: forward flexion, hyperextension, lateral bending, rotation.			
M. Hips			
1. Hips for symmetry and level of gluteal folds.			
2. Palpate hips and pelvis for instability, tenderness, and crepitus.			
3. Test range of motion: flexion, extension, and hyperextension; adduction; abduction; internal and external rotation.			
4. Test muscle strength: knee in flexion and extension, abduction and adduction.			
N. Legs and knees			
1. Knees for natural concavities			
2. Palpate the popliteal space and joint space			
3. Test range of motion: flexion and extension			
4. Test the strength of muscles in flexion and extension			
O. Feet and ankles			
1. Feet and ankles during weight bearing and non–weight bearing for contour, alignment with tibias, size, number of toes.			
2. Palpate the Achilles tendon and each metatarsal joint			
3. Test range of motion: dorsiflexion and plantar flexion, inversion and eversion, and flexion and extension of the toes.			
4. Test strength of muscles in plantar flexion and dorsiflexion.			

| | Assessed Appropriately by Student? | | Comments |
	Yes	No	
I. Inspection, palpation, and neurologic tests			
A. Test cranial nerves I through XII.			
1. I (olfactory)			
2. II (optic)			
3. III (oculomotor)			
4. IV (trochlear)			
5. V (trigeminal)			
6. VI (abducens)			
7. VII (facial)			
8. VIII (acoustic)			
9. IX (glossopharyngeal)			
10. X (vagus)			
11. XI (spinal accessory)			
12. XII (hypoglossal)			
B. Cerebellar function and proprioception			
1. Evaluate coordination and fine motor skills by rapid rhythmic alternating movements, accuracy of upper and lower extremity movements.			
2. Evaluate balance using the Romberg test.			
3. Observe the patient's gait for posture and rhythm and sequence of stride and arm movements.			
C. Sensory function			
1. Test primary sensory responses to superficial touch and pain.			
2. Test vibratory response to tuning fork over joints or bony prominences on upper and lower extremities.			
3. Evaluate perception of position sense with movement of the great toes or a finger on each hand.			
4. Assess ability to identify familiar object by touch and manipulation.			
5. Assess two-point discrimination.			

Continued

193

	Assessed Appropriately by Student?		Comments
	Yes	No	
6. Assess ability to identify letter or number "drawn" on palm of hand.			
7. Assess ability to identify body area when touched.			
D. Superficial and deep tendon reflexes			
1. Test abdominal reflexes.			
2. Test the cremasteric reflex in male patients.			
3. Test the plantar reflex.			
4. Test the following deep tendon reflexes: biceps, brachioradialis, triceps, patellar, and Achilles.			
5. Test for ankle clonus.			

	Performed Appropriately by Student?		Comments
	Yes	No	
I. At the start of the interview			
A. Say "hello" and greet the patient appropriately.			
B. Introduce self and ask others present how they are related to the patient.			
C. Give appropriate attention to everyone's comfort.			
D. Eliminate noise and other distractions when possible.			
E. Outline the purposes of the interview and assess the patient's understanding.			
F. Begin with a comfortable, open-ended question, such as, "How can I be of help?"			
II. During the interview			
A. Encourage and facilitate further response, (e.g., with a head nod).			
B. Follow responses to open-ended questions with appropriate specific questions.			
C. Consistently seek clarification when a response was in some way unclear.			
D. Direct the course of the interview gently.			
E. Ask one question at a time.			
F. Occasionally restate what was heard to check accuracy.			
III. Throughout the interview			
A. Maintain appropriate eye contact.			
B. Maintain a comfortable posture, invoking body language that shows attentiveness to the patient.			
C. Use appropriate silence, allowing enough time for the patient's comments, expressions, thoughts, and feelings.			
D. Empathize when appropriate.			
E. Restate willingness to help when appropriate.			
F. Confirm being the patient's ally in working together to find appropriate outcomes.			
G. Ensure that the patient has the necessary understandings.			
IV. At the close of the interview			
A. Summarize and recheck for accuracy.			
B. Ask if there are any other questions or concerns.			
C. Appropriately indicate next steps.			
D. Say "thank you" with appreciation and with an appropriate "good-bye."			

	Assessed Appropriately by Student?		Comments
	Yes	No	
I. General medical history			
A. Illnesses or injuries since the previous health visit or PPE			
B. History of having been denied or restricted from participation in sporting activities and reason for restriction			
C. History of heat illness or muscle cramps			
D. Current viral illness			
E. Sickle cell trait or disease			
F. Hospitalizations or surgeries			
G. All medications used by the athlete			
H. Use of any special equipment or protective devices during sports participation			
I. Allergies			
J. Absence of paired organs			
K. Immunization status, including hepatitis B, varicella, meningococcal, human papillomavirus, and pertussis			
L. Height, weight, and body mass index (BMI)			
M. Palpation of lymph nodes			
II. Cardiac			
A. Symptoms of exertional chest pain/discomfort			
B. Unexplained syncope or near syncope			
C. Excessive exertional and unexplained dyspnea or fatigue, associated with exercise			
D. Prior recognition of a heart murmur			
E. Elevated systemic blood pressure			
F. Family history of premature death			
G. Family history of disability from heart disease in a close relative younger than 50 years			
H. Specific knowledge of certain cardiac conditions in family members: hypertrophic or dilated cardiomyopathy, long-QT syndrome or other ion channelopathies, Marfan syndrome, or clinically important arrhythmias			
I. Heart rate and rhythm to assess for arrhythmias, heart murmur			
J. Femoral pulses to exclude coarctation of the aorta			
K. Physical stigmata of Marfan syndrome			
L. Brachial artery blood pressure			

Continued

Chapter **Student Performance Checklists**

	Assessed Appropriately by Student?		Comments
	Yes	No	
III. Respiratory			
A. Coughing, wheezing, or dyspnea with exercise			
B. Previous use of asthma medications			
C. Family history of asthma			
D. Lung auscultation			
IV. Neurologic			
A. History of a head injury with or without symptoms of a concussion			
B. Numbness or tingling in the extremities			
C. Headaches			
D. History of seizure			
E. History of inability to move an extremity after a collision			
V. Vision			
A. Visual problems			
B. Glasses or contact lenses			
C. Previous eye injuries			
D. Visual acuity			
VI. Orthopedic			
A. Previous injuries that have limited sports practice or participation			
B. Injuries that have been associated with pain, swelling, or the need for medical intervention			
C. Previous fractures or dislocated joints			
D. Previous or current use of a brace, orthotic, or other assistive device			
E. Screening orthopedic examination			
VII. Psychosocial			
A. Weight control and body image			
B. Dietary habits; calcium intake			
C. Stresses in personal life, at home, or in school			
D. Feelings of sadness, hopelessness, depression or anxiety			
E. Use or abuse of recreational drugs, alcohol, tobacco, dietary or performance supplements			
F. Attention to signs of eating disorders, including oral ulcerations, decreased tooth enamel, edema			

	Assessed Appropriately by Student?		Comments
	Yes	No	
VIII. Genitourinary and abdominal			
A. Age at menarche, last menstrual period, regularity of menstrual periods, number of periods in the last year, and longest interval between periods			
B. Palpation of the abdomen for organomegaly			
C. Palpation of the testicles			
D. Examination for inguinal hernias			
IX. Dermatologic			
A. A. History of rashes, pressure sores, or other skin conditions			
B. History of boils or MRSA skin infections			
C. Skin lesions suggestive of HSV, MRSA, or tinea corporis			

Answer Key

CHAPTER 1

Terminology Review

1. Cultural knowledge
2. Cultural humility
3. Genomics
4. Culture
5. Cultural desire
6. Culturally competent care
7. Cultural awareness
8. Stereotype
9. Precision Medicine
10. Cultural skill

Application to Clinical Practice

Clinical Case Study

1. Need for an interpreter
2. What do you call your problem?
   What do you think caused your problem?
   Why do you think it started when it did?
   What does your sickness do to you?
   How does it work?
   How bad is your sickness?
   How long do you think it will last?
   What should be done to get rid of it?
   Why did you come to me for treatment?
   What benefit will you get from treatment?
   What are the most important problems your sickness has caused for you?
   What worries you and frightens you the most about your sickness?
   Who else or what else might help you get better?
   Has anyone else helped you with this problem?
3. "I know there are traditional Chinese ways of treating sickness."
   "Do you know any of them? What are they?"
   "Have you tried any of them for your pain?"
   "Did they help?"
4. Cereal grains and chili peppers

Concepts Application

Term	Definition
Gender-diverse	Person whose gender identity differs from that sex assigned at birth but may be more complex or fluid. It can encompass individuals who identify as non-binary, genderqueer, gender fluid and a host of other descriptors.
Sexual orientation	A person's sexual, romantic, emotional, physical attraction towards other people.
Transgender	Person whose gender identity differs from sex assigned at birth
Gender/gender identity	A person's internal sense of self and how they fit into the world from the perspective of gender.
Nonbinary	Not identifying as exclusively male or female within the traditional gender binary of Western European-based culture
Sex	Sex assigned at birth, historically based on a cursory visualization of external genitalia.

Critical Reasoning

Clinical Reasoning Case Study 1

1. A transgender man is a person with a male gender identity and a female birth assigned sex.
2. "Cold" foods include cod fish and fresh vegetables; "cold" medicines and herbs the patient might have tried include orange flower water and soda.

Clinical Reasoning Case Study 2

1. *Health belief and practices:* What does illness mean to you? How do you perceive your health? What do you currently do to treat your illness and to help you stay healthy?
2. *Religious and ritual influences:* Do you have any special religious practices or beliefs? Are there any special practices you follow or beliefs you have about illness or dying?

201

3. *Dietary practices:* What does your family eat? Who prepares the food? How is the food prepared?
4. *Family relationships:* What are the roles of your family members? Who is responsible for child rearing?

Self Reflection

If you are unsure of your responses, please review the components of a cultural response in your textbook.

Content Review Questions

Multiple Choice

1. d
2. d
3. c
4. d
5. a
6. b
7. b
8. c
9. a
10. c
11. b
12. d
13. a
14. b

CHAPTER 2

Terminology Review

1. Intimate partner violence (IPV)
2. Symptom analysis

3. CAGE
4. Family history (FH)
5. Chief concern (CC)
6. Personal and social history (SH)
7. Functional assessment
8. Past medical history (PMH)
9. History of present illness (HPI)
10. Review of systems (ROS)

Application to Clinical Practice

Clinical Case Study

1. The chief complaint is fatigue.
2. Questions to ask:
   When did the fatigue start?
   What does it feel like?
   How often does it occur?
   What factors have made it improve or get worse?
   How severe is the fatigue?

3. Goal of the Review of Systems (ROS) is to identify presence or absence of health issues in each of the body systems.
4. Questions to be asked during the ROS relate to general and constitutional symptoms, skin, head, neck, eye, ear, nose, mouth and throat, lymph nodes, chest and lungs, breasts, heart and blood vessels, peripheral vasculature, hematologic status, gastrointestinal system, diet, endocrine system, musculoskeletal system, nervous system, genitourinary function, and psychiatric problems.

Concepts Application

Patient Behavior Issue	Examiner Behavior to Decrease Tension
Seduction	Do not respond to seductive behavior. Be courteous, calm, firm, and direct from the start. Send the message that the relationship is, and will remain, professional.
Depression	Do not ignore it. Gather information about the patient's feelings. Do not hurry the patient. Avoid superficial reassurance.
Anxiety	Avoid overload of information. Pace the conversation and maintain a calm demeanor.
Excessive flattery	Be aware that this is possibly a manipulation on the part of the patient; it is easy to be taken in by such manipulations.
Financial concerns	Be aware that the patient may be concerned about the cost of healthcare; be prepared to talk about it with the patient.
Silence	Be patient. Allow a moment of silence. Silence allows the patient a moment of reflection.

Clinical Reasoning

Clinical Reasoning Case Study 1

1. O (onset)—started 2 weeks ago
   L (location)—outside edge of the heel of the left foot
   D (duration)—lasts 2 to 3 hours in the morning
   C (characteristic)—burning pain
   A (aggravating factors)—walking barefoot
   R (relieving factors)—ice and Tylenol one to two times per day
   T (timing)—upon awakening
   S (severity)—severe pain

Clinical Reasoning Case Study 2

1. Components of a health history present in the case study:
   CC
   HPI
   ROS
   PMH
   SH

2. The FH should have been added to the health history.
3. Components that are only partially complete:
   ROS—additional head and neck and reproductive questions
   SH—living situation questions

Patient Safety Consideration

You might consider breaking the confidentiality of patient–healthcare provider communication when information is shared that suggests a patient or other person may be at risk for injury.

Application to Clinical Practice

Clinical Concepts Application 1

Description	Examination Technique or Equipment
Gathering information through touch	Palpation
Used to assess for macular degeneration	Amsler Grid
Measures percentage of hemoglobin saturated with oxygen	Pulse oximetry
Source of light with a narrow beam	Transilluminator
Used to test deep tendon reflexes	Percussion hammer
Used to visualize turbinates	Nasal speculum
Assesses near vision	Rosenbaum or Jaeger chart
Tests for loss of protective sensation in the skin	Monofilament
Larger field of view in eye examination	Pan-optic ophthalmoscope

Content Review Questions

Multiple Choice

1. c
2. c
3. b
4. c
5. d
6. a
7. b
8. b
9. a
10. c
11. c
12. a
13. c
14. c
15. b
16. d
17. d
18. d
19. a
20. b

CHAPTER 3

Terminology Review

1. Percussion
2. Bell of stethoscope
3. Goniometer
4. Amsler grid
5. Tuning fork
6. Stadiometer
7. Ophthalmoscope
8. Aperture setting
9. Otoscope
10. Transilluminator
11. Doppler
12. Tympanometer
13. Diaphragm of stethoscope
14. Snellen chart
15. Wood's lamp

203

Clinical Concepts Application 2

Area Percussed	Percussion Tone Expected
Stomach	Tympanic
Sternum	Flat
Lung of patient with emphysema	Hyperresonant
Liver	Dull
Lung of patient with pneumonia	Dull
Lung of normal patient	Resonant
Abdomen with large tumor	Dull

Clinical Reasoning

Clinical Reasoning Case Study 1

1. Place the patient in a separate room. Wear gloves for the examination. Properly dispose of any disposable items that come into contact with the patient. Disinfect the room and all nondisposable articles after the patient leaves.

Clinical Reasoning Case Study 2

a. Remove the speculum and take the patient's blood pressure.
b. Sweating or goose bumps, blotchy skin, nausea, and severe high blood pressure are signs of autonomic hyperreflexia, a potentially life-threatening problem occurring in patients with spinal cord injuries at T6 or higher. It is triggered by stimulation of the bowel, bladder, or skin below the level of the injury.

Patient Safety Consideration

It is important to know your own strength because you need to know when to call for assistance if a patient needs help with activities such as transferring or getting on the examination table. Calling for assistance when needed protects both the patient and the examiner from injury.

Content Review Questions

Multiple Choice

1. c	3. d
2. d	4. b

Application to Clinical Practice

Concepts Application

Symptoms	Body Systems That Might Be Involved
Chest pain	Cardiovascular, respiratory, musculoskeletal
Headaches	Neurologic, cardiovascular, visual, auditory
Abdominal pain	Cardiovascular, gastrointestinal, urinary
Pain in the legs	Musculoskeletal, neurologic, integumentary, cardiovascular

5. b	16. d
6. a	17. c
7. a	18. a
8. a	19. c
9. d	20. d
10. a	21. a
11. c	22. a
12. b	23. c
13. a	24. a
14. c	25. d
15. b	26. d

CHAPTER 4

Terminology Review

1. False negative
2. Clinical reasoning
3. Negative predictive value
4. Sensitivity
5. Bayes formula
6. True negative
7. Evidence-based practice (EBP)
8. Behavior change
9. True positive
10. Occam's razor
11. Specificity
12. False positive
13. Positive predictive value
14. Autonomy
15. Nonmaleficence

Matching

1. b
2. c
3. d
4. a

Critical Thinking

Matching

1. c
2. g
3. d
4. a
5. f
6. b
7. e

Concepts Application

Examination Data	Possible Problems
A 54-year-old woman with jaundice, abdominal pain, nausea, and weight loss. Has pain with abdominal palpation; positive bowel sounds. Liver slightly enlarged; admits to alcohol use.	Cholecystitis, hepatitis, pancreatitis, cirrhosis, hepatic malignancy
A 66-year-old man with a chief complaint of breathing difficulty. Has increased respiratory rate, low-grade fever, rales, productive cough; increased tactile fremitus bilaterally.	Pneumonia, pulmonary edema, empyema
A 13-week-old infant girl with fever, irritability, poor eating. Infant is dehydrated and has a temperature of 103.7°F; soft abdomen.	Otitis media, upper respiratory infection, gastroenteritis
A 19-year-old female college student with a chief complaint of pain when urinating. Describes frequency and urgency. Patient has temperature of 100.4°F; has constant pain in pelvic area; positive pain with fist percussion over left flank.	Urinary tract infection, pyelonephritis, sexually transmitted infection

Content Review Questions

Multiple Choice

1. a
2. c
3. d
4. c
5. b
6. d
7. c
8. a
9. c
10. a

9. Past medical history
10. History of present illness
11. Family history
12. Problem list

Application to Clinical Practice

Concepts Application 1

1. Subjective
2. Chief concern
3. SOAP
4. Illustration
5. Objective
6. Incremental grading
7. POMR
8. Health history
9. Physical examination

CHAPTER 5

Terminology Review

1. Problem-oriented medical record (POMR)
2. Episodic illness visit
3. OLDCARTS mnemonic
4. Information integrity
5. Chief concern
6. Personal and social history
7. Plan
8. Comprehensive health history and physical examination

Concepts Application 2

Problem #	Onset	Problem	Date Resolved
1.	January 2021	Low back pain	Ongoing
2.	2005	IDDM—poor control	Ongoing
3.	May 2001	Cholecystitis	Resolved
4.		Family history of ASHD	Ongoing
5.		Family history of CRF	Ongoing

205

Case Study

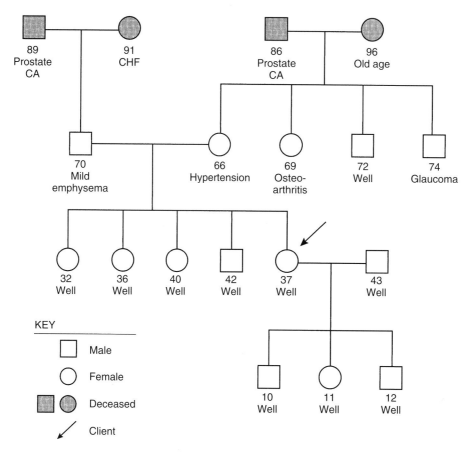

KEY

☐ Male

◯ Female

▨ ⬤ Deceased

↙ Client

Clinical Reasoning

1. "OLDCARTS" refers to the following: O = onset of symptom; L = location of the symptom; D = duration of the symptom; C = character of the symptom; A = aggravating or associated factors of the symptom; R = relieving factors; T = temporal factors; and S = severity of the symptom.

2. Organs, masses, and lesions should be documented based on the following characteristics: texture or consistency; size; shape or configuration; mobility; tenderness; induration; heat; color; location; and other characteristics, such as bleeding, discharge, and scarring.

Patient Safety Consideration

When documenting in a patient record, two major ways to contribute to meeting The Joint Commission patient safety goal of improved communication among caregivers are to (1) avoid using abbreviations and (2) use CPCF selectively and with great care.

Content Review Questions

Multiple Choice

1. a
2. d
3. c
4. b
5. d

6. a
7. c
8. c
9. a
10. c

CHAPTER 6

Terminology Review

1. Tachypnea
2. Pyrexia
3. Blood pressure (BP)
4. PAINAD
4. Neonatal Infant Pain Scale
6. Neuropathic pain
7. Temperature
8. Complex regional pain syndrome
9. FLACC Behavioral Pain Assessment Scale
10. Pulse rate
11. Korotkoff sounds
12. Respiratory rate
13. Wong/Baker faces rating scale
14. Shivering
15. Pulse pressure

Application to Clinical Practice

Clinical Case Study 1

1. Date of onset, duration, cyclic nature, variability, related to injury or exposure to illness

2. *Associated symptoms:* Sweating, chills, irritability, nausea, vomiting, fatigue

3. *Medications:* Acetaminophen or nonsteroidal antiinflammatory drugs

206

Clinical Case Study 2

Diagnosis	Pain Findings
Acute pain	Vital sign changes, pallor, diaphoresis, dry mouth, facial mask of pain, irritability
Carpal tunnel syndrome	Burning, shocklike pain
Colitis	Cramping, guarding over abdomen
Osteoarthritis	Tender, deep, and aching pain

Clinical Reasoning

Clinical Reasoning Case Study 1

1. Stiffness of blood vessels and increased vascular resistance
2. Increased vagal tone

Clinical Reasoning Case Study 2

1. Guarding of the abdomen, change in vital signs, facial distortions, dry mouth, pupil dilation
2. Visceral or colic pain

Patient Safety Consideration

The plan calls for you to assess the patient at the time of peak effect of the analgesic. This addresses patient safety because patients should be checked at this time not only for effectiveness of pain relief but also for the occurrence of deleterious effects, some of which may be life threatening.

Content Review Questions

Multiple Choice

1.	a	11.	a
2.	d	12.	a
3.	b	13.	c
4.	c	14.	c
5.	a	15.	a
6.	b	16.	a
7.	b	17.	b
8.	b	18.	a
9.	a	19.	b
10.	d	20.	c

CHAPTER 7

Terminology Review

1. Insults
2. Coherence
3. Wernicke
4. Apraxia
5. Dysphonia
6. Affect
7. Glasgow Coma Scale
8. Broca
9. Aphasia
10. Judgment
11. Cognitive
12. Dysarthria
13. Comprehension
14. Hallucination

Application to Clinical Practice

Matching

1.	d	4.	a
2.	b	5.	c
3.	f	6.	e

Clinical Concepts Application

1. *Attention:* Recite a list of numbers slowly and have the patient repeat them in the correct order. The patient should be able to repeat the series of numbers correctly.
2. *Recent Memory:* Give the patient a short time to view four or five test objects, saying that you will ask about the objects in a few minutes. Ten minutes later, ask the patient to list the objects. All objects should be remembered.
3. *Judgment:* Ask the patient hypothetical questions involving situations in which decisions must be made, such as finding money on the sidewalk or seeing a car on fire. The patient should be able to evaluate a situation and describe an appropriate action to take in the circumstances.
4. *Abstract reasoning:* Recite a common proverb to the patient and request an explanation of its meaning. The patient should be able to give appropriate interpretations within one's cultural frame of reference.
5. *Thought processes and content:* Observe the patient's pattern of thought during the interview and examination process. The patient should be logical, coherent, and goal oriented.

Clinical Case Study

1. *Data deviating from normal:* The patient recently lost her spouse. Son says his mother has "gone downhill." Son indicates patient is no longer keeping her house clean or cooking appropriate meals. Son reports significant change in patient's personal hygiene habits. Son reports that patient becomes angry when he talks about other living options. Patient states, "You think I am helpless and want to lock me away." Patient is a 78-year-old woman who sits quietly during conversation. Overall hygiene is clean, but her hair is matted, and her clothes are wrinkled and do not match. Overall affect is very dull; she makes no eye contact with her son or the examiner.

207

2. The examiner should ask additional questions related to the behaviors cited as concerns by her son. Such question would include the following: "What is meant by not cooking appropriate meals?" and "In what way is the house not clean?" The patient herself should be asked about her daily diet and if there is a reason for the changes in her living patterns. Other questions should be aimed at gathering more information about cognitive abilities and emotional stability. These could include questions about ability to shop and pay the cashier, manage a checking account, increasing difficulty remembering recent events, or coming up with the right name for things. Given the recent loss of her spouse, questions screening for depression and suicide potential may be asked.

3. The examiner should conduct a physical examination that will provide clues to her cognitive abilities as well as her emotional stability. Screening tests for dementia and depression should be done. Physical assessment focused on nutritional status and skin condition as problems in these areas could result from inappropriate meals and poor personal hygiene.

4. The patient may have depression.

Clinical Reasoning

1. **Depression** is associated with grief, a stressful life event, a reaction to medical or neurologic diseases, or a change in lifestyle. It may occur suddenly or slowly and is characterized by impaired concentration, reduced attention span, indecisiveness, slower thought processes, and impaired short- and long-term memory. The patient often feels sad, hopeless, and worthless and has a loss of interest or pleasure, but there are no delusions or hallucinations. Insomnia or excessive sleeping, fatigue, restlessness, anxiety, and increased or decreased appetite may also occur. Depression can be treated and it can recur.

   Delirium may be associated with infections, medications, electrolyte and metabolic disorders, major organ failure, brain insults, and acute alcohol withdrawal; it lasts for hours or days. It is characterized by a sudden onset, altered consciousness; impaired memory, attentiveness, and consciousness; rapid mood swings; rambling and illogical or incoherent speech; and increased or decreased activity. Misperceptions, illusions, hallucinations, and delusions are common. Delirium may be reversible.

   Dementia, associated with a structural disease of the brain, is characterized by a slow, persistent, and progressive course that cannot be reversed. Initially, the patient has minimal cognitive impairment. As the disorder progresses, abstract thinking, judgment, memory, thought patterns, and calculations become impaired. Delusions may be present, but misperceptions and hallucinations are usually absent. Speech may become rambling and

incoherent as the patient struggles to find words. Behavior is usually unchanged.

2. Cognitive function should remain intact. Decreases in speed of information processing and psychomotor speed accompanied by less cognitive flexibility are expected but no decline in the ability to plan and develop strategies, organize, concentrate and remember details, and manage activities (executive functioning) should occur.

Patient Safety Consideration

Implement patient safety monitoring and obtain an immediate psychiatry referral.

Content Review Questions

Multiple Choice

1.	d	6.	b
2.	d	7.	c
3.	b	8.	b
4.	a	9.	b
5.	c	10.	c

CHAPTER 8

Terminology Review

1. Velocity
2. Macronutrients
3. Pica
4. Sexual maturity rating
5. Ballard gestational age assessment
6. Head circumference
7. Waist-to-height ratio
8. Body mass index
9. Micronutrients
10. Gestational age
11. Recumbent length
12. Failure to thrive
13. Obesity
14. Twenty-four-hour recall

Application to Clinical Practice

Clinical Case Study 1

1. Current BMI = 21.08
2. Previous BMI = 25.55

Personal Food Record
Answers will vary.

Personal Food Assessment
Answers will vary.

Personal Analysis of Nutritional Needs
Answers will vary.

Clinical Reasoning

1. a. *Growth hormone:* Secreted by the pituitary gland; promotes growth and increase in organ size, and regulates carbohydrate, protein, and lipid metabolism.
   b. *Growth hormone–releasing hormone (GHRH):* Stimulates the pituitary to release growth hormone.
   c. *Somatostatin:* Inhibits secretion of both GHRH and thyroid-stimulating hormone.
   d. *Insulin-like growth factor (IGF-I):* In conjunction with growth hormone, stimulates muscle and skeletal growth.
2. a. *Sex steroids (androgens):* Stimulate increased secretion of the growth hormone, which mediates the increase in IGF-I.
   b. *Testosterone:* Enhances muscular development and sexual maturation; promotes bone maturation and epiphyseal closure.
   c. *Estrogen:* Stimulates development of secondary sex characteristics and skeletal maturation
3. Leptin has a key role in regulating body fat mass; Its concentration is thought to be a trigger for puberty by informing the central nervous system that adequate nutritional status and body fat mass are present to support pubertal changes and growth.

Matching
1. f
2. c
3. e
4. d
5. b
6. a

Patient Safety Consideration
Answers will vary.

Content Review Questions

Multiple Choice
1. d
2. b
3. b
4. c
5. b
6. d
7. b
8. c
9. d
10. a
11. d
12. a
13. d
14. b
15. a

Clinical Concepts Application

Type of Lesion	Examples
1. Excoriation	Abrasion, scratch, scabies
2. Fissure	Athlete's foot, cracks at corner of mouth
3. Erosion	Varicella or variola after rupture
4. Ulcer	Pressure ulcers, stasis ulcers

CHAPTER 9

Terminology Review
1. Annular
2. Confluent
3. Generalized
4. Nevus
5. Vesicle
6. Acrocyanosis
7. Lanugo
8. Petechiae
9. Morbilliform
10. Alopecia
11. Telangiectasias
12. Chloasma
13. Salmon patches (stork bites)
14. Ecchymosis
15. Sebum
16. Plaque
17. Dermatomal
18. Keloid
19. Stellate
20. Melanin
21. Vernix caseosa
22. Reticulate
23. Serpiginous

Application to Clinical Practice

Anatomy Review
a. Cuticle
b. Nail plate
c. Perionychium
d. Lunula
e. Eponychium

Matching 1

1. c	6. i
2. h	7. a
3. e	8. f
4. g	9. b
5. d	

Matching 2

1. d	3. c
2. b	4. a

Matching 3

1. a	5. b
2. b	6. c
3. a	7. a
4. a	8. c

Clinical Case Study

1. All data described are considered normal for the age of the patient, with the exception of the ulcerations on the lower extremities. This could be caused by a number of factors, but it is definitely not within normal limits for any age.
2. Ask when he first noticed the lesions, how often he has had the lesions, and what seems to help them get better. Ask if he has any pain in his legs associated with activity.
3. Assess circulation to the feet. An ulcerated open wound that does not heal most likely indicates insufficient perfusion of blood, leading to tissue anoxia. It is possible that a Doppler study may be needed to assess pulses or vascular studies may need to be considered.
4. The most common reason for this problem is insufficient perfusion. This may be the result of underlying vascular disease or heart disease; it may also be associated with diabetes.

Clinical Reasoning

1. Explain the early signs of melanoma to the patient using the ABCDE guideline:

   A = Asymmetry. Melanoma lesions are asymmetric in shape and appearance.

   B = Border. Melanoma lesions have irregular, indistinct, and sometimes notched borders.

   C = Color. Melanoma lesions tend to have uneven and variegated color. Lesions may vary from brown to pink to purple or have a mixed pigmentation.

   D = Diameter. Melanoma lesions are usually greater than 6 cm (size of a pencil eraser) in diameter.

   E = Evolution. Changes seen in existing pigmented lesions, particularly in a nonuniform, asymmetric manner can indicate melanoma

2. The examiner should note the following: location (where the lesion is found), distribution (isolated lesions or confluent), color, size, pattern (clustered, linear), shape, elevation (flat, raised), and characteristics (hard, soft, crusty, fluid-filled, solid, draining).

Patient Safety Consideration

How did he get his deep tan? Does he work outside? Does he spend leisure time in the sun? Does he use sunscreen and, if so, what SPF and how much and how often does he apply it? Does he know the risks associated with sun exposure? Does he practice regular skin self-examination?

Content Review Questions

Multiple Choice

1. a	11. a
2. c	12. a
3. a	13. a
4. b	14. b
5. d	15. c
6. c	16. d
7. c	17. d
8. d	18. b
9. b	19. c
10. a	20. d

CHAPTER 10

Terminology Review

1. Shotty nodes
2. Lymph
3. Lymphangioma
4. Acute suppurative lymphadenitis
5. Lymphadenopathy
6. Lymphangitis
7. Lymphedema
8. Fluctuant
9. Matted
10. Lymphadenitis

Application to Clinical Practice

Anatomy Review

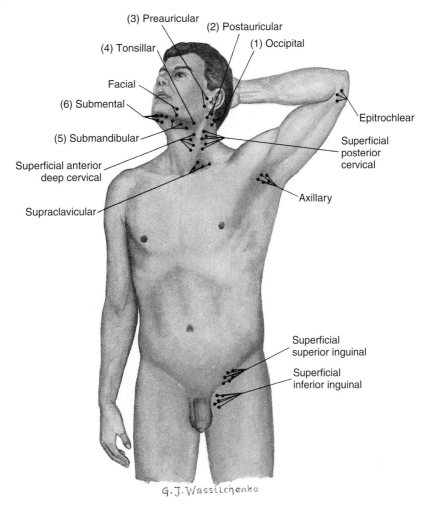

(3) Preauricular
(2) Postauricular
(4) Tonsillar
(1) Occipital
Facial
(6) Submental
Epitrochlear
(5) Submandibular
Superficial posterior cervical
Superficial anterior deep cervical
Axillary
Supraclavicular
Superficial superior inguinal
Superficial inferior inguinal

G.J.Wassilchenko

Matching

1. i
2. c
3. h
4. a
5. d

6. g
7. f
8. b
9. e

Clinical Case Study

1. Data deviating from normal: Fatigue and weakness, enlarged lymph nodes
2. Ask whether there is tenderness to the lymph nodes. Ask whether the patient has been ill recently. Ask whether he has had recent weight loss, has been eating properly, and has been getting adequate sleep.
3. Assess lymph nodes in neck, axilla, arm, and groin. Compare palpable lymph nodes for symmetry. Note the size, consistency, mobility, borders, and tenderness of lymph nodes.

4. Enlarged lymph nodes could be the result of a recent viral infection or a more serious problem such as a lymphoma or malignancy.

Clinical Reasoning

1. Compared with that of an adult, the lymph system of an infant or small child is proportionally much larger (the thymus, in particular, is quite large). Lymph nodes are normally readily palpable. After puberty, the lymph nodes become small and much less pronounced. The thymus shrinks to a point where it is not assessed. By the time an adult reaches late adult years, the lymph nodes become very small and have limited function. The nodes become fibrotic and fatty and become impaired in their ability to resist infection.

Content Review Questions

Multiple Choice

1.	a	11.	d
2.	d	12.	d
3.	b	13.	b
4.	d	14.	a
5.	b	15.	c
6.	b	16.	c
7.	c	17.	d
8.	c	18.	a
9.	a	19.	c
10.	d	20.	d

CHAPTER 11

Terminology Review

1. Mastoid fontanel
2. Chloasma
3. Plagiocephaly
4. Facies
5. Webbing
6. Bulging fontanel
7. Microcephaly
8. Bruit
9. Torticollis
10. Encephalocele
11. Molding
12. Ossification
13. Craniosynostosis
14. Exophthalmos
15. Macewen sign
16. Tic

Application to Clinical Practice

Matching

1.	d	4.	e
2.	c	5.	b
3.	a		

Anatomy Review

a. Hyoid bone
b. External carotid artery
c. Thyroid cartilage
d. Internal jugular vein
e. Common carotid artery
f. Thyroid gland
g. Right subclavian artery
h. Right subclavian vein
i. Brachiocephalic artery and vein
j. Internal carotid artery
k. Carotid sinus
l. Pyramidal lobe (thyroid gland)
m. Trachea
n. Lymph node
o. External jugular vein
p. Left subclavian artery
q. Left subclavian vein
r. Arch of aorta

Concepts Application

System or Structure	Hyperthyroidism	Hypothyroidism
Weight	Weight loss	Weight gain
Emotional state	Nervous; irritable	Lethargic; disinterested
Temperature preference	Prefers cool climate	Prefers warm climate
Hair	Fine hair with hair loss	Coarse hair that breaks easily
Skin	Warm skin with hyperpigmentation	Coarse, dry, scaling skin at pressure points
Neck	Goiter	No goiter
Gastrointestinal	Increased peristalsis; increased frequency of bowel movements	Decreased peristalsis; constipation
Eyes	Proptosis (exophthalmos); lid retraction	Puffiness in periorbital region

Case Study

1. Data deviating from normal: Patient complains of severe recurring headache. Nasal stuffiness occurs with headache. Nothing seems to help headache.
2. Get more information about the headache, including the following:
   Pattern of headaches: How often do the headaches occur? At what time of day do they occur? How would you characterize the onset of the headaches (gradual vs. sudden)?
   Characteristics of headache: Where is the pain? What is the pain like? How long does the pain last? How severe is the pain?
   Precipitating factors: What brings the headache on?
   Treatment: What has been done to try to treat these headaches?

212

History: Is there any past or recent history of trauma to the head?

3. Assess range of motion in the neck, if possible, and attempt to palpate the neck for lymph nodes.

Clinical Reasoning

1. Percussion of the head and neck is not routinely performed. One exception is when evaluating for hypocalcemia, percussion on the masseter muscle may produce a hyperactive masseteric reflex; the Chvostek sign.
2. Similar to percussion, auscultation of the head is not routinely performed. However, if a vascular anomaly of the brain is suspected, bruits might be heard. It is best to listen over the eyes, the temporal region, and just below the occiput of the skull.

Patient Safety Consideration

"Back to Sleep" positioning reduces the incidence of sleep-related infant death. Infants can develop a flattened head from lying in one position, but the risk can be reduced by alternatingleft and right supine head position starting at birth and by supervised, awake tummy time.

CONTENT REVIEW QUESTIONS

Multiple Choice

1. c		9. d	
2. b		10. b	
3. d		11. d	
4. d		12. a	
5. a		13. c	
6. b		14. d	
7. d		15. a	
8. a			

CHAPTER 12

Terminology Review

1. Presbyopia
2. Ectropion
3. Lipemia retinalis
4. Pterygium
5. Anisocoria
6. Drusen bodies
7. Glaucomatous optic nerve cupping
8. Band keratopathy
9. Hemianopia
10. Ptosis
11. Hordeolum
12. Adie pupil (tonic pupil)
13. Xanthelasma
14. Entropion
15. Nystagmus
16. Strabismus
17. Argyll Robertson pupil
18. Cotton wool spot
19. Hypertelorism
20. Papilledema
21. Miosis
22. Mydriasis
23. Red reflex

Application to Clinical Practice

Matching 1

1. c	4. a
2. b	5. d
3. e	6. f

Concepts Application 1

Structure	What Should Be Examined
1. Eyelid	Observe position of the eyelids when the eyes are open and when the eyelids are closed completely. Inspect for eversion or inversion of the eyelids and the presence of nodules.
2. Conjunctiva	Inspect for inflammation, presence of foreign body, and increased erythema or exudate. Observe for pterygium.
3. Cornea	Assess corneal sensitivity. Note lipid deposits on cornea. Assess clarity.
4. Iris and pupil	Check for response to light and accommodation. Estimate pupillary sizes; compare them for equality.
5. Lens	Inspect for clarity—lens should appear transparent.
6. Sclera	Check for color of sclera and for pigmentation.
7. Lacrimal apparatus	Inspect and palpate. Check for tearing.

213

Concepts Application 2

1. a. Location: Lesion is 2 DD at clock position of 2:00
   b. Length: 2/3 DD
   c. Width: 1/3 DD

Matching 2

1. c	4. b
2. d	5. e
3. a	

Case Study

1. Data deviating from normal: History of poorly controlled diabetes; change in vision; significant visual acuity findings; ophthalmoscope findings; new vessels and presence of hemorrhage vessels
2. Ask the patient whether he has pain. Ask if the change in vision has been gradual and progressive and if it is constant or intermittent. Ask about other symptoms associated with the change in vision, such as intolerance to light. Ask him whether he currently wears contact lenses or glasses. Ask how long he has had diabetes.
3. It is important to determine the previous visual acuity results to compare with the current results.
4. There is one major problem at this point that affects multiple areas. If he loses his vision, the impact on functional abilities will be tremendous and will include (but not be limited to) safety, self-care activities, management of his diabetes, independence, and employment.

Clinical Reasoning

1. General inspection of external structures of the eye should be done. Visual acuity should be checked with a Snellen chart. A red reflex should be checked; corneal light and reflex and cover–uncover should also be done. Finally, examination of extraocular movements and cranial nerves III, IV, and VI should be done, including asking the child to follow through the six cardinal fields of gaze.
2. The first clue is the size; retinal arteries are about one-third narrower than retinal veins. The second difference is the color. Arteries appear as a very light red color. Veins, on the other hand, are darker in color.

Patient Safety Consideration

1. Only if there is a need to evaluate for retinal disease.
2. Inspect the patient's anterior chamber by shining a focused light tangentially at the limbus. If the nasal portion of the iris is not lighted, the patient has a shallow anterior chamber and is at risk for acute-angle glaucoma.

Content Review Questions

Multiple Choice

1. d	11. a
2. b	12. a
3. c	13. d
4. b	14. b
5. a	15. b
6. c	16. b
7. a	17. c
8. c	18. b
9. b	19. a
10. c	20. d

CHAPTER 13

Terminology Review

1. Rinne test
2. Frenulum
3. Xerostomia
4. Otosclerosis
5. Conductive hearing loss
6. Cerumen
7. Weber test
8. Fordyce spots
9. Sensorineural hearing loss
10. Epstein pearls
11. Torus
12. Ossicles
13. Cheilitis
14. Epistaxis
15. Presbycusis
16. Vertigo

Application to Clinical Practice

Matching

1. c	6. i
2. b	7. h
3. d	8. f
4. a	9. e
5. g	

Anatomy Review

a. Auricle
b. External auditory canal
c. Tympanic membrane
d. Stapes and footplate
e. Eustachian tube
f. Round window
g. Oval window
h. Cochlea
i. Cochlear and vestibular branches of the auditory nerve
j. Facial nerve
k. Semicircular canals
l. Incus
m. Malleus

Clinical Application

1. Koplik spots
2. Darwin tubercle
3. Malocclusion
4. Epstein pearls

Case Study

1. Data deviating from normal: Fever; complaints of ear pain; presence of drainage in ear canal; tympanic membrane perforation; reduction of hearing in left ear; flat affect; limited talking.
2. Ask what treatment the child has received for the ear pain from the medicine man in the past. Ask the mother whether she has ever seen drainage from the ear with past problems. Ask whether the child has been treated at a hospital or clinic for ear pain in the past.
3. If possible, complete a Rinne test. A full hearing assessment with an audiometer is probably in order as well. Also, complete a developmental assessment.
4. Primary problems: The child has obvious ear disease. There is also some evidence of a possible developmental delay, perhaps associated with the hearing loss.

Clinical Reasoning

1. To differentiate redness associated with crying versus otitis media, look for other clinical signs, primarily bulging and mobility of the tympanic membrane.

Patient Safety Consideration

The auditory canal is easily abraded, causing pain and bleeding; therefore, a cerumen spoon must be used with care.

Generally, irrigation with water at body temperature is the preferred method of cerumen removal in young patients.

Water irrigation is contraindicated if the patient has an infection of the external auditory canal, pressure-equalizing tubes, perforated tympanic membrane, or an opening into the mastoid.

Content Review Questions

Multiple Choice

1. a	9. b
2. c	10. d
3. b	11. b
4. a	12. b
5. d	13. d
6. c	14. c
7. c	15. a
8. a	

CHAPTER 14

Terminology Review

1. Wheeze
2. Egophony
3. Pectoriloquy
4. Cheyne-Stokes respiration
5. Vocal resonance
6. Stridor
7. Apnea
8. Fine crackles
9. Bronchovesicular breath sounds
10. Kussmaul breathing
11. Biot respirations
12. Rhonchi
13. Crackles
14. Tracheomalacia
15. Bronchophony
16. Coarse crackles
17. Hamman sign
18. Medium crackles
19. Pleural friction rub
20. Vesicular breath sounds

Application to Clinical Practice

Auscultation Sounds

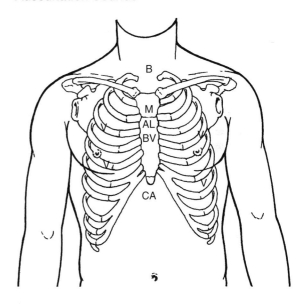

Examination Technique

Finding	Examination Method	Finding	Examination Method
Biot respiration	Inspection	Bronchial	Auscultation
Tactile fremitus	Palpation	Rhonchi	Auscultation
Cheyne-Stokes respiration	Inspection	Barrel chest	Inspection
Dullness	Percussion	Hyperresonance	Percussion
Vesicular	Auscultation	Wheezes	Auscultation
Tympany	Percussion	Tracheal tug	Palpation
Dyspnea	Inspection	Crackles	Auscultation
Bronchophony	Auscultation	Diaphragmatic excursion	Percussion
Vibration	Palpation	Bronchovesicular	Auscultation
Kussmaul breathing	Inspection	Crepitus	Palpation or auscultation

Matching

1. d
2. j
3. h
4. g
5. b
6. i
7. f
8. c
9. e
10. a

Case Study

1. Data deviating from normal: History of shortness of breath; limitation in activity; interrupted sleep (requiring pillows); smoking history; labored breathing with tachypnea; presence of cyanosis; underweight with protruding ribs; increased anteroposterior diameter; reduced chest wall movement; diminished tactile fremitus; adventitious breath sounds; diminished breath sounds.
2. Ask about chest pain with shortness of breath. Ask about the presence of cough. Ask how old the patient was when she started smoking and how long she has been smoking as much as she currently is.
3. Assess oxygen saturation, body weight, and rhythm of breathing pattern. Assess for presence of retractions. Percuss the chest for tone and diaphragmatic excursion.
4. Primary problems for this patient include respiratory or oxygenation problems and nutrition problems. Patients who are short of breath have difficulty maintaining adequate nutrition.

Clinical Reasoning

1. He has a 9-year history of one-third pack a day (3 pack years), a 15-year history of half a pack a day (7½ pack-years), and a 32-year history of 1 pack a day (32 pack-years) for a total of a 42½ pack-year history.
2. These symptoms are consistent with tuberculosis. High-risk groups include Native Americans or American Indians and immigrants from Mexico. He should be placed in airborne isolation until a diagnosis is made.

3. Ask what has changed. The mother said the family moved recently; ask about the new home and environment as well as possible irritants within the new home. Also ask about ventilation, air conditioning, and exposure to smoke and pets in or around the home.

Patient Safety Consideration

The upper airway is severely obstructed when
- stridor is inspiratory and expiratory.
- cough has a barking character.
- retractions also involve the subcostal and intercostal spaces.
- cyanosis is obvious even with supplemental oxygen.

Content Review Questions

Multiple Choice

1. d
2. c
3. d
4. a
5. c
6. a
7. c
8. d
9. c
10. a
11. b
12. a
13. c
14. b
15. d
16. b
17. d
18. a
19. d
20. a

CHAPTER 15

Terminology Review

1. Sinoatrial node
2. Point of maximal impulse (PMI)
3. Intrinsic
4. Thrill
5. Purkinje fibers
6. Diastole
7. Atria

8. Heave
9. Regurgitation
10. Pericardium
11. Still murmur
12. Pulmonic valve
13. Myocardium
14. Septum
15. Systole

c. Coronary sulcus
d. Right coronary artery
e. Right atrium
f. Anterior cardiac veins
g. Right ventricle
h. Apex
i. Left ventricle
j. Left coronary artery
k. Great cardiac vein
l. Left atrium
m. Left pulmonary artery
n. Arch of aorta
o. Left subclavian artery
p. Left common carotid artery

Application to Clinical Practice

Anatomy Review

a. Brachiocephalic artery
b. Superior vena cava

Concepts Application

Valve	Where Would You Auscultate?
Tricuspid valve	Fourth intercostal space at left sternal border
Mitral valve	Fifth intercostal space at left midclavicular line
Aortic valve	Second right intercostal space at left sternal border
Pulmonic valve	Second left intercostal space at left sternal border

Matching

1. g
2. i
3. c
4. d
5. e
6. j
7. a
8. h
9. b
10. f

Case Study

1. Data deviating from normal: Shortness of breath; fatigue that interferes with routine activities; sleeping difficulty; labored breathing with elevated respiratory rate, pulse rate, and blood pressure; pitting edema in lower extremities; frothy-looking phlegm.
2. Complete a symptom analysis on the shortness of breath and fatigue. Ask the patient whether he has symptoms associated with chest pain, cough, or nocturia. Ask the patient about cardiovascular history.
3. Perform a precordial assessment, including inspection, percussion, palpation, and auscultation.
4. First, this patient has a perfusion problem. The decrease in cardiac output reduces the transport of oxygenated blood throughout the body. Second, this patient has an oxygenation problem. Because the heart is not pumping efficiently, blood is backing up in the pulmonary bed, resulting in pulmonary edema. Pulmonary edema interferes with the exchange of oxygen and carbon dioxide in the lungs. Fatigue results from impaired tissue oxygenation.

Clinical Reasoning

1. This finding, without other symptoms, may not be relevant. However, children who have congenital heart defects tend to squat frequently because squatting relieves dyspnea.
2. Look for polyarthritis, chorea, erythema marginatum, subcutaneous nodules, arthralgia, an increase in the sedimentation rate, and leukocytosis.
3. Diabetes causes an increase in the basement membrane of capillaries, which makes these vessels narrower. Narrowing contributes to hypertension and impaired perfusion of the lower extremities.

Patient Safety Consideration

Say "Sit up slowly" when the patient is getting up from a lying position on the examining table.
Have the patient sit with legs dangling for a minute before getting off the examining table.
Be ready to provide assistance if needed when the patient changes position.

Content Review Questions

Multiple Choice

1. c
2. b
3. a
4. a
5. c
6. c
7. c
8. b
9. b
10. c
11. c
12. a
13. c
14. a
15. b
16. d
17. d
18. a
19. d
20. d

CHAPTER 16

Terminology Review

1. Varicose veins
2. Hum
3. Jugular pulse wave
4. Claudication
5. Venous thrombosis
6. Arterial embolic disease
7. Raynaud phenomenon
8. Venous ulcers
9. Bruit
10. Pitting
11. Arteriovenous fistula
12. Arterial aneurysm
13. Peripheral arterial disease
14. Regurgitation

Application to Clinical Practice

Anatomy Review

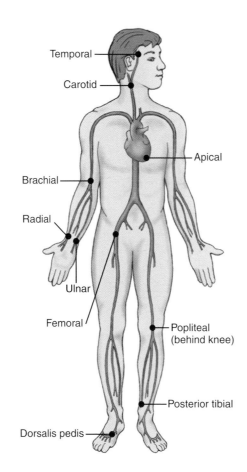

From Bonewit-West K, Hunt SA, Applegate E. *Today's Medical Assistant: Clinical & Administrative Procedures*, 3rd ed. St. Louis, MO: Elsevier, 2016.

Concepts Application 1

Location of Pain	Probable Obstructed Artery
Calf muscles	Superficial femoral artery
Thigh	Common femoral artery or external iliac artery
Buttock	Common iliac artery or distal aorta

Concepts Application 2

Arterial Insufficiency	Venous Insufficiency or Musculoskeletal Disorders
1. Pain comes on during exercise.	Pain comes on during or often several hours after exercise.
2. Pain is quickly relieved by rest.	Pain is relieved by rest but sometimes only after several hours or even days. Pain tends to be constant.
3. Intensity of pain increases with intensity and duration of exercise.	Intensity of pain has greater variability than arterial pain in response to intensity and duration of exercise.

Matching

1. d   5. h
2. e   6. g
3. b   7. a
4. c   8. f

Case Study

1. Data deviating from normal: Changes in color and temperature of the hands; exertional dyspnea; presence of dark lesion on the fifth right finger
2. Complete a symptom analysis on the circulation in the hands and the dyspnea. Ask the patient whether the pain and color changes vary with activity or environmental changes; also, ask how long the episodes of pain last and how frequently they occur. Ask the patient about other symptoms of dyspnea that may be interfering with activities of daily living.
3. Perform further neurologic assessment of the hands; obtain chest film and pulmonary function studies; complete evaluation for connective tissue disease, including appropriate laboratory work (ESR, ANA titer, and chemistry studies).
4. This patient has a circulatory problem that is most likely secondary to connective tissue disease and exacerbated by smoking. The intermittent spasms of the arterioles in the fingers cause pallor, and the accompanying decrease in circulation produces claudication. The appearance of impending ulceration on the finger signals the need for monitoring of the patient's circulatory status. The patient may develop spasms in the nose and tongue. The patient should be educated about this possibility and encouraged to report any changes in her circulatory status.

Clinical Reasoning

1. The symptoms suggest venous thrombosis, and the patient is at risk for pulmonary embolus.
2. Blood pressure can change with position changes by the mother. Hypotension is frequently noted during the third trimester when the patient is supine. This is secondary to venous occlusion of the vena cava and resulting impaired venous return. In addition, blood tends to stagnate in the lower extremities as a result of occlusion of the pelvic veins and the inferior vena cava caused by the growing uterus.

Patient Safety Consideration

When palpating the carotid arteries, never palpate both sides simultaneously. Excessive carotid sinus massage can cause slowing of the pulse, a drop in blood pressure, and compromised blood flow to the brain, leading to syncope.

Content Review Questions

Multiple Choice

1. c   11. a
2. b   12. c
3. a   13. a
4. c   14. b
5. b   15. c
6. c   16. a
7. b   17. d
8. c   18. b
9. b   19. c
10. d   20. b

CHAPTER 17

Terminology Review

1. Thelarche
2. Cooper ligaments
3. Montgomery follicles
4. Virchow nodes
5. Fat necrosis
6. Tail of Spence
7. Areola
8. Gynecomastia
9. Mammogram
10. Tanner staging
11. Galactorrhea
12. Duct ectasia
13. Colostrum
14. Involution
15. Peaud'orange appearance

Application to Clinical Practice

Matching

1. d   5. c
2. e   6. h
3. b   7. g
4. a   8. f

219

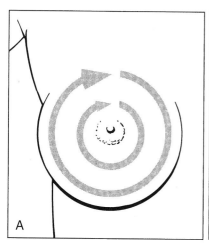 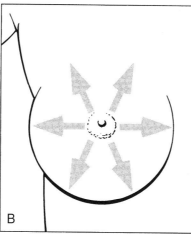 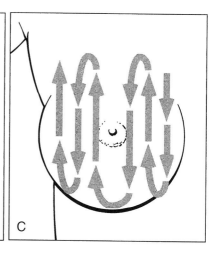

A B C

Case Study

1. Data deviating from normal: Patient has a history of a nontender breast lump, noticeable for about 9 months. Mass has increased in size over 9 months. Risk factors include early onset of menarche and the fact that the patient is childless. Palpable lump is present in the left upper outer quadrant. Dimpling noted on left breast. Left nipple is retracted. Bloody discharge is noted from nipple when squeezed.

2. Ask about personal or family history of breast disease. Ask the patient whether she does regular breast self-examinations. Ask whether she has ever had a mammogram. Ask about location of the lump. Ask whether the lump is tender now. Ask whether she has noticed nipple discharge. Ask about changes in the lump size in relation to her menstrual cycle.

3. Inspect the areola. Besides location, the following characteristics must be assessed with a breast mass: size, shape, consistency, tenderness, mobility, and borders. Palpate the axilla. It is especially important to note any lumps or masses in the left axilla.

4. Primary problems: This patient has a very suspicious breast mass consistent with malignancy. She also seems to be in denial about this problem.

Clinical Reasoning

1. Risk factors for breast cancer: Patient is female. She is older than 40 years of age. She had an early onset of menarche. She had her first and only child at the age of 36 years. She has a strong family history of breast cancer. Although it cannot be predicted who will and will not develop breast cancer, this woman certainly has very strong risk factors.

2. Information on breast screening guidelines:
   - Breast cancer screening recommendations for women at average risk vary by authority.
   - Issues regarding screening recommendations are the ages at which to start and stop screening, the screening interval (annual vs. biennial), and the screening modality (clinical breast examination [CBE], mammography, and tomosynthesis [creates a three-dimensional view], alone or in combination).
   - Evidence from the systematic reviews performed by the U.S. Preventive Services Task Force and the American Cancer Society shows that breast cancer mortality is reduced with mammography screening, although estimates are of borderline statistical significance. Most of the benefit of mammography results from screening during ages 50 to 74 years.
   - Breast cancer screening involves a trade-off of benefits and potential harms.
   - Screening decisions should be made in the context of informed shared decision-making.

Content Review Questions

Multiple Choice

1.	d	10.	d
2.	c	11.	b
3.	a	12.	a
4.	c	13.	b
5.	c	14.	a
6.	c	15.	b
7.	b	16.	a
8.	d	17.	d
9.	b	18.	c

CHAPTER 18

Terminology Review

1. Colic
2. Striae
3. Scaphoid abdomen
4. Mesentery
5. Pylorus
6. Peristalsis
7. Borborygmi
8. Tympany
9. Reflux
10. Hydronephrosis
11. Peritoneum
12. Ballottement
13. Pepsin
14. Ascites
15. Intussusception
16. Renal calculi

Application to Clinical Practice

Anatomy Review

a. Liver
b. Gallbladder
c. Ascending colon
d. Small intestine
e. Cecum
f. Appendix
g. Bladder
h. Sigmoid colon
i. Descending colon
j. Transverse colon
k. Stomach
l. Spleen

Matching 1

1. d	4. e
2. c	5. f
3. a	6. b

Concepts Application 1

Structure	Quadrant	Region
Appendix	Right lower quadrant	Right inguinal
Colon	Ascending or transverse right upper quadrant	Ascending—right lumbar
	Transverse and descending left upper quadrant	Transverse—umbilical
	Ascending right lower quadrant, descending left lower quadrant	Descending—left lumbar
Gallbladder	Right upper quadrant	Right hypochondriac
Liver	Right upper quadrant	Right hypochondriac (right lobe) Epigastric
Pancreas	Left upper quadrant (body)	Epigastric
	Right upper quadrant (head)	Left hypochondriac (tail)
Small intestine	Right lower quadrant	Umbilical
	Left lower quadrant	Hypogastric
Spleen	Left upper quadrant	Left hypochondriac
Stomach	Left upper quadrant	Left hypochondriac

Concepts Application 2

Condition	Type of Pain	Abdominal Signs	Associated Symptoms or Findings
Peritonitis	Sudden or gradual onset of generalized or localized pain described as dull or severe; increased pain with deep inspiration	+ Markle sign + Balance sign + Blumberg sign	Shallow respirations; nausea and vomiting; guarding; decreased bowel sounds; + obturator and iliopsoas tests
Cholecystitis	RUQ and epigastric pain that refers to right subscapular region	+ Murphy sign	Anorexia, vomiting, fever, right upper quadrant tenderness and rigidity
Ectopic pregnancy	Lower quadrant pain that may refer to the shoulder; agonizing pain with rupture	+ Cullen sign + Kehr sign	Symptoms of pregnancy, spotting, hypogastric tenderness, mass on bimanual pelvic examination; with rupture: shock, rigid abdominal wall distention
Pancreatitis	Sudden and dramatic LUQ, umbilical, or epigastric pain that may be referred to left shoulder	+ Grey-Turner sign + Cullen sign	Fever, epigastric tenderness, vomiting
Renal calculi	Intense flank pain extending to groin and genitals	+ Kehr sign	Fever, hematuria

Concepts Application 3

Sounds of Auscultation	Possible Associated Condition
Increased bowel sounds	Gastroenteritis, early intestinal obstruction, or hunger
High-pitched tinkling sounds	Intestinal fluid and air under pressure, as in early obstruction
Decreased bowel sounds	Peritonitis and paralytic ileus
Friction rub	Inflammation of the peritoneal surface from tumor, infection, or infarction
Venous hum	Increased collateral circulation between portal and systemic venous systems

Matching 2

1. e
2. h
3. c
4. i
5. g
6. d
7. a
8. j
9. f
10. b

Case Study

1. Data deviating from normal: Abdominal pain (progressively worse); loss of appetite and nausea; guarded position; hot skin, possibly indicating fever; absence of bowel sounds; pain on palpation and guarding RLQ; positive rebound tenderness in RLQ.
2. Ask the patient about vomiting with her nausea. Ask about her menstrual cycle, about the possibility of pregnancy, and about bowel elimination and the appearance of her stool.
3. Check vital signs (of particular interest is temperature). Auscultate for arterial bruits and venous hums. Percuss kidney for costovertebral angle tenderness. Perform iliopsoas muscle test and obturator muscle test.
4. Primary problems: Patient demonstrates symptoms consistent with acute abdominal condition, very likely appendicitis. A complete blood count would be helpful.

Clinical Reasoning

1. Listen to the abdomen for bruits in the aortic, renal, iliac, and femoral arteries. A bruit in these arteries may indicate stenosis or an aneurysm. Listen in the umbilical area for a venous hum (soft, low pitched, and continuous). A venous hum suggests increased collateral circulation between portal and systemic venous systems and may indicate portal hypertension. A friction

rub is high pitched and may be heard in association with respiration. This may indicate inflammation of the peritoneal surface from tumor or infection.

2. Ask Mr. Cane to place his hand on top of his abdomen. You will then place one of your hands on the side of his abdomen near the flank; use the other hand to tap on the other side of the abdomen. The test result is considered positive if the tap causes a fluid wave through the abdomen that is felt by your hand on the side of his abdomen.

3. Expected findings unique to pregnancy include decreased bowel sounds, linea nigra, striae, diastasis recti, quickening, and venous pattern.

Patient Safety Consideration

Be very gentle when palpating for the spleen. Patients with splenomegaly from mononucleosis have an increased risk of splenic rupture. Related advice on confirmation of mononucleosis would be to avoid risk of trauma to the area of the spleen, such as by avoiding contact sports for 6 weeks.

Content Review Questions

Multiple Choice

1. d	12. d
2. c	13. a
3. c	14. a
4. a	15. c
5. d	16. a
6. b	17. b
7. c	18. a
8. c	19. a
9. d	20. b
10. d	21. c
11. b	22. d

CHAPTER 19

Terminology Review

1. Atrophic vaginitis
2. Hydrocolpos
3. Chadwick sign
4. Rectouterine pouch
5. Uterine prolapse
6. Caruncle
7. Menarche
8. Bartholin glands
9. Infertility
10. Rectocele
11. Hegar sign
12. Ambiguous genitalia
13. Cystocele
14. Mittelschmerz
15. Skene ducts

Application to Clinical Practice

Anatomy Review

a. Prepuce
b. Labium minus
c. Hymen
d. Vaginal orifice
e. Vestibule
f. Fourchette
g. Anus
h. Mons pubis
i. Clitoris
j. Urethral or urinary orifice
k. Labium majus
l. Bartholin duct opening
m. Perineum

Matching 1

1. O, E
2. C
3. O, E
4. C
5. C
6. E
7. C, O, E
8. C

Matching 2

1. d	5. g
2. e	6. b
3. a	7. c
4. f	

Concepts Application

Position	Description	Advantages or Disadvantages
Knee–chest	Patient lies on side with both knees bent, with top leg closer to chest.	Does not require stirrups. Good position for patients who feel comfortable and balanced in a side-lying position.
Diamond shape	Patient lies on back with knees bent so that legs are spread flat and heels meet at the foot of the table.	Patient must be able to lie flat on back for this position and have flexible legs.
Obstetric stirrups	Patient lies on back near foot of the table with legs supported under the knees in obstetric stirrups.	These offer more support than the traditional foot stirrups. Patient may need help positioning legs in stirrups.
M-shape	Patient lies on back, knees bent apart, feet resting on the examination table close to buttocks.	Entire body can be supported by the table.
V-shape	Patient lies on back with legs straightened out and spread wide to either side of the table.	Patient must be able to lie comfortably on the back. Assistance is needed to maintain this position.

Case Study

1. Data deviating from normal: History suggests some type of acute inflammation. History is also suggestive of multiple sex contacts; primary partner has multiple sex contacts. Mass with inflammation, discharge, and extreme pain on palpation needs further evaluation.
2. Ask patient about sexual history and associated medical problems, if any. Identification of protection (or lack of) would also be helpful.
3. A culture of discharge should be obtained for evaluation. If the patient is too uncomfortable for internal examination, this may need to be delayed until the inflammation has resolved.
4. Based on symptoms and findings, the patient most likely has an acute abscess of the Bartholin gland. This is frequently associated with gonococcal or staphylococcal infection.

Clinical Reasoning

1. The key concept when performing an examination on a patient with a visual impairment is to explain everything that is to occur and what you want the patient to do. Before the examination, the patient should be given an opportunity to explore the instruments used during the examination. Other general concepts to keep in mind include introducing yourself, remembering to identify others who enter the room, and letting the patient know when others are leaving the room. Also, orient the patient to the surroundings. This patient may need assistance in getting into the proper position for examination.
2. The history is vital to obtain. At this age, it is necessary to talk with her while her parents are out of the room. Questions should be simple, gentle, and nonjudgmental. These will greatly improve the accuracy of the information she is willing to share. There is no one set rule to determine the age when a full examination of the genitalia is necessary. However, a good rule of thumb is that if the patient is sexually active, then an examination should be done. The examination should be carried out similarly to that of an adult.

Patient Safety Consideration

As you withdraw the speculum, the blades will tend to close themselves; thus care must be taken to avoid pinching the cervix and vaginal walls. Maintain downward pressure of the speculum to avoid trauma to the urethra. Hook your index finger over the anterior blade as it is removed. Keep one thumb on the handle lever and control closing of the speculum. Make sure that the speculum is fully closed when the blades pass through the hymenal ring.

Content Review Questions

Multiple Choice

1. c	11. a
2. a	12. d
3. b	13. d
4. b	14. b
5. a	15. c
6. b	16. c
7. c	17. a
8. d	18. c
9. b	19. d
10. b	20. c

CHAPTER 20

Terminology Review

1. Phimosis or paraphimosis
2. Chordee
3. Spermatocele
4. Glans
5. Priapism
6. Hydrocele
7. Adhesions
8. Escutcheon
9. Testicular torsion
10. Varicocele
11. Cryptorchidism
12. Cremasteric
13. Hypospadias
14. Peyronie

Application to Clinical Practice

Anatomy Review

a. Rectum
b. Seminal vesicle
c. Levator ani muscle
d. Ejaculatory duct
e. Anus
f. Bulbocavernosus muscle
g. Epididymis
h. Glans
i. Testis
j. Urethra
k. Corpus spongiosum
l. Corpus cavernosum
m. Prostate gland
n. Symphysis pubis
o. Urinary bladder

Matching 1

1. d
2. b
3. e
4. a
5. c

Matching 2

1. c
2. d
3. a
4. b
5. e

Case Study

1. Data deviating from normal: Protrusion or mass is noted in left groin area. History suggests a possible hernia.
2. Discuss the patient's level of discomfort and other related symptoms. Determine whether there is history of this problem.
3. Examiner needs to determine whether this hernia is reducible. If it is nonreducible, it may require prompt surgical intervention. Also, full examination of the genitalia is in order.
4. Based on symptoms and findings, the patient most likely has a direct inguinal hernia.

Clinical Reasoning

1. Discuss the role of genital self-examination in identifying sexually transmitted infections. Discuss how to perform genital self-examination. This should include the following: inspection of the tip for evidence of swelling, sores, or discharge; palpation of the entire shaft of the penis from the base to the glans to feel for lumps or tenderness; and examination of the scrotum for color, texture, and presence of lesions.
2. Be sure one of the child's parents is present. Explain to the child what you must do and why (to be sure all his body parts are healthy). It may be necessary for the parent to reassure the child that it is OK for the examiner to see his "privates."

Patient Safety Consideration

Binding adhesions may develop as a result of forceful retraction of the foreskin.

Content Review Questions

Multiple Choice

1. d
2. c
3. c
4. b
5. b
6. c
7. a
8. c
9. a
10. a
11. c
12. d
13. a
14. d
15. b
16. c
17. a
18. a
19. c
20. d

CHAPTER 21

Terminology Review

1. Prostate gland
2. Hemorrhoids
3. Anal fistula
4. Rectum
5. Imperforate anus
6. Enterobiasis (roundworm or pinworm)
7. Pruritus ani
8. Anal canal
9. Rectal prolapse
10. Pilonidal cyst
11. Anorectal fissure
12. Polyp

Application to Clinical Practice

Anatomy Review 1

a. Superior rectal valve
b. Internal hemorrhoidal plexus
c. Internal sphincter
d. Superficial external sphincter
e. Anal crypt

f. Subcutaneous external sphincter
g. Perianal gland
h. Rectal sinus
i. Rectal column
j. Deep external sphincter
k. Levator ani muscle
l. Inferior rectal valve
m. Middle rectal valve

Anatomy Review 2

a. Prostate gland
b. Utricle
c. Opening of Cowper gland
d. Cowper gland
e. Ejaculatory orifice

Matching

1. b	5. a
2. f	6. e
3. d	7. c
4. g	

Case Study

1. Data deviating from normal: Sensation of rectal full-ness; rectal bleeding; blood in stool; palpable mass in the rectum; weight loss; enlargement of prostate.
2. Ask the patient about changes in bowel elimination pattern or changes in the appearance of the stools (besides presence of blood). Ask about abdominal discomfort or distention. Ask about problems with urination (problems with starting or force of stream). Ask about sexual history.
3. Examination should include guaiac test and inguinal lymph node assessment. As part of the abdominal assessment, the examiner should specifically consider the possibility of pelvic or abdominal masses.
4. The patient has an enlarged prostate and a rectal mass. They may be interrelated or completely independent of one another. Further diagnostic testing is indicated.

Clinical Reasoning

1. The symptoms have some similarity, but findings will be different.
   Acute prostatitis: The patient will have an inflamed prostate; therefore, the prostate will be tender, and the patient will likely have a fever. Symptoms of obstruction develop more quickly than with the other two problems. With palpation, the prostate will be tender and possibly asymmetric. Additionally, the seminal vesicles may be dilated and tender to palpation.
   Benign prostate hypertrophy: Symptoms will develop gradually, with complaints of hesitancy, decreased force of stream, dribbling, and incomplete empty-ing of the bladder. With palpation, the prostate will feel rubbery, symmetric, and enlarged.
   Prostatic carcinoma: The symptoms of obstruction gradually occur. With palpation, the prostate is hard and irregular and feels asymmetric; the median sulcus is obliterated.

2. Some of the questions you could ask include:
   When did bleeding start?
   How much bleeding have you noticed?
   When and where do you see the bleeding?
   What does the blood look like?
   Do you have any other symptoms associated with the bleeding, such as pain, gas, cramping, or weight loss?
   What do you think is causing the bleeding?

Patient Safety Consideration

When examining the position and patency of a neonate's anus, care must be taken not to confuse a perianal fistula with an anal orifice.

Content Review Questions

Multiple Choice

1. a	11. b
2. b	12. c
3. b	13. d
4. d	14. d
5. a	15. c
6. a	16. d
7. b	17. b
8. d	18. c
9. a	19. a
10. c	20. d

CHAPTER 22

Terminology Review

1. Pronation
2. Scoliosis
3. Dislocation
4. Inversion
5. Muscle strain
6. Eversion
7. Adduction
8. Supination
9. Dupuytren contracture
10. Gower sign
11. Polydactyly
12. Gibbus
13. Goniometer
14. Abduction
15. Crepitus
16. Kyphosis
17. Syndactyly

Application to Clinical Practice

Matching 1

1. e	6. d
2. b	7. a
3. h	8. g
4. b	9. c
5. f	10. e

Concepts Application 1

Symptoms and Assessment Findings	Problems to Consider
Heberden nodes and Bouchard nodes noted on hands	Osteoarthritis
Low back pain that radiates to the buttocks and posterior thigh, with tenderness over the spine	Lumbar disk herniation
Heat, redness, swelling, and tenderness to the metatarsophalangeal joint	Gouty arthritis of the great toe
Subcutaneous nodules on the forearm near the elbow	Rheumatoid arthritis
Tenderness, swelling, and a boggy sensation with palpation along the grooves of the olecranon process; increased pain with pronation and supination	Epicondylitis or tendonitis
A child with muscle atrophy and symptoms of progressive muscle weakness	Muscular dystrophy
A child complaining of pain in the elbow and wrist; will not move his or her arm; maintains arm in a flexed and pronated position	Radial head subluxation

Matching 2

1. f
2. b
3. g
4. h
5. c
6. d
7. a
8. e

Case Study

1. Data deviating from normal: Diagnosis of RA; significant joint pain; limitations in self-care activities; limitations in socialization; difficulty with posture and gait; deformities to joints; tender, inflamed joints with palpation; subcutaneous nodules at the ulnar surface of the elbows.
2. Ask the patient what medications she is taking for the RA. Find out whether she is involved with any other nonpharmaceutical therapies. Ask her whether these things help or make a difference. Ask whether she has any assistive devices that she uses or whether she receives any assistance with self-care activities.
3. The examiner should perform documentation of ROM in various joints. Use of a goniometer would be particularly helpful.
4. Self-care activities, pain, social isolation

Clinical Reasoning

1. Muscle strain results if a muscle is stretched or torn beyond its functional capacity. A sprain is a stretching or tearing of a supporting ligament of a joint. A fracture is a partial or complete break in the continuity of the bone. Because the injury involves the joint, muscle strain is not likely. Both fractures and sprains are associated with pain and swelling and can have a bluish discoloration, so it is not always easy to differentiate these. If the patient is able to walk bearing weight on the affected ankle, it is doubtful that a fracture resulted; if he was unable to bear weight at all, it could be a fracture or a severe sprain. Thus, radiography is usually the final diagnostic indicator.

2. A dislocation of the radial head, or radial head subluxation, is caused by jerking the arm upward while the elbow is flexed. This can occur by someone pulling on a child's arms during play or even while dressing a child. The parents must understand how this injury occurred and be taught to avoid arm-pulling activities.

Patient Safety Consideration

Safety needs of all patients regardless of type of problem are similar. Every patient needs to get the right care, at the right time and in the right way. Every patient needs protection against accidental harm related to equipment and environmental hazards. However, the patient with a musculoskeletal problem is likely to have special needs related to support, stability, and movement, which are the functions of the musculoskeletal system. Of course, any patient may have a musculoskeletal problem concomitant with the problem that prompted a healthcare visit. Thus, careful attention to a patient's limitations and need for assistance is always an essential component of care, especially critical for the patient seeking care for an acute musculoskeletal problem that interferes with stability and mobility.

Content Review Questions

Multiple Choice

1. a
2. b
3. c
4. d
5. c
6. d
7. d
8. a
9. b
10. c
11. c
12. a
13. c
14. a
15. b
16. d
17. c
18. b
19. b
20. c

227

CHAPTER 23

Terminology Review

1. Lower motor neuron disorder
2. Kernig sign
3. Occipital lobe
4. Basal ganglia
5. Temporal lobe
6. Stereognosis
7. Cerebellum
8. Normal-pressure hydrocephalus
9. Shaken baby syndrome
10. Pseudotumor cerebri
11. Ataxia
12. Nuchal rigidity
13. Thalamus
14. Antalgic
15. Steppage gait
16. Hypothalamus
17. Graphesthesia
18. Brainstem
19. Romberg sign
20. Brudzinski sign
21. Frontal lobe
22. Medulla oblongata

Application to Clinical Practice

Anatomy Review 1

a. Pituitary gland
b. Optic chiasma
c. Hypothalamus
d. Corpus callosum
e. Cerebrum
f. Skin
g. Superior sagittal sinus
h. Thalamus
i. Skull
j. Dura mater
k. Galea aponeurotica
l. Tentorium cerebelli
m. Midbrain
n. Cerebellum
o. Pons
p. Medulla oblongata

Anatomy Review 2

a. Cerebrum
b. Thalamus
c. Hypothalamus
d. Cerebral peduncle
e. Cerebellum
f. Hypoglossal (XII)
g. Spinal accessory (XI)
h. Vagus (X)
i. Glossopharyngeal (IX)
j. Acoustic (VIII)
k. Facial (VII)
l. Abducens (VI)
m. Trigeminal (V)
n. Trochlear (IV)
o. Oculomotor (III)
p. Pituitary gland
q. Optic (II)
r. Olfactory (I)

Concepts Application 1

Examination Procedure	Cranial Nerve(s) Tested
Whisper test	CN VIII
Patient sticks out tongue and moves it toward nose and toward chin	CN XII
Taste test with sugar, salt, and lemon	CN VII (anterior), CN IX (posterior)
Visual acuity	CN II
Patient puffs out cheeks and shows teeth	CN VII
Patient shrugs shoulders against examiner's hands	CN XI
Smell test with coffee, orange, and cloves	CN I
Pupils constrict and dilate in response to light	CN III
Patient clenches teeth (temporal muscles contracted)	CN V

Concepts Application 2

Age of Infant	Observed Response	Name of Reflex	Expected or Unexpected?
2 months	The infant demonstrates a strong grasp of the examiner's finger when it is placed in the infant's palm.	Palmar grasp	Expected; this should disappear by 3 months.
4 months	When held in an upright position with the soles of the feet touching the surface of a table, the infant flexes the legs upward in a curled position and holds them there.	Stepping	Unexpected; although the age is appropriate, the expected observed response is an alternating flexion and extension of the legs.
6 months	With the child lying supine, turn the head to one side; the arm and leg extend on the side that the head was turned toward.	Asymmetric tonic neck	Unexpected at 6 months.
8 months	The infant abducts and extends the arms and legs in response to sudden movement of the head and trunk backward. The arms then adduct in an embracing motion, followed by relaxation.	Moro	Unexpected; this should disappear by 6 months of age.

Matching

1. c
2. b
3. g
4. e
5. a
6. h
7. d
8. f
9. i

Case Study

1. Data deviating from normal: Patient has been diagnosed with CVA. He had a headache preceding the incident. Patient's history includes inability to talk. He has left-sided paresis. He requires assistance for mobility. Patient avoids eye contact and cries.
2. Ask the patient whether he thinks he can swallow normally. Ask him whether he has any pain or discomfort. Ask the patient's wife about her husband's medical and family history. Ask about medications her husband may be currently taking. Ask whether her husband lost consciousness or had a seizure with this incident.
3. Assess gag reflex. Test reflexes (deep tendon). Assess for drooling.
4. Patient has weakness on one side of his body, which affects nearly all aspects of functional abilities. He has problems with communication, nutrition, and mobility as well.

Clinical Reasoning

1. The examiner's findings are invalid because he did not adjust his tool to determine two-point discrimination. Different body surfaces have varying sensitivity; depending on what body surface is being tested, the distance between two points on the tool must be adjusted. For instance, on the fingertips, the minimal distance for the two points is 2.8 mm. On the chest and forearms, the minimal distance is 40 mm. Most body surfaces are not able to detect one point versus two points at 1 inch (2.5 mm) apart.
2. The frontal lobe is the primary motor cortex; thus, an infarction in this area will affect motor function primarily on the opposite side of the lesion. Because the patient has a left infarction, he will be affected on the right side. Additionally, if the Broca area is affected, the motor dysfunction will affect this patient's ability to form words.

Patient Safety Consideration

1. The examiner needs to be prepared to catch the patient should the patient fall.
2. If the patient has a positive Romberg sign, the examiner should postpone other tests of cerebellar function that require balance.

Content Review Questions

Multiple Choice

1. c
2. a
3. b
4. d
5. c
6. b
7. a
8. b
9. c
10. d
11. d
12. d
13. a
14. c
15. a
16. a
17. a
18. a
19. d
20. b

CHAPTER 24

Terminology Review

1. Language barriers
2. Activities of daily living (ADLs)
3. Sensory deprivation
4. Emotional constraints, apparent and inapparent
5. Basic activities of daily living
6. Functional assessment
7. Instrumental activities of daily living
8. Cultural barriers

Application to Clinical Practice

Matching

1. f		10. l	
2. j		11. d, e	
3. h		12. m	
4. e		13. j	
5. k		14. i	
6. m		15. m	
7. b, c		16. f	
8. g		17. j	
9. a		18. m	

Concepts Application

Examination Area	Body Systems Examined
Upper extremities	Integumentary, cardiovascular, respiratory, lymphatic, musculoskeletal, neurologic
Anterior chest	Integumentary, cardiovascular, respiratory, lymphatic, musculoskeletal, breasts and axillae
Abdomen	Integumentary, gastrointestinal, cardiovascular, musculoskeletal, lymphatic, neurologic
Head and neck	Integumentary, lymphatic, neurologic, musculoskeletal, visual, auditory, nose and paranasal, mouth and oropharynx

Clinical Reasoning

1. The most significant modification necessary with this examination is communication. It is vital that the examiner explain what is to be done and how. Even though a visual acuity examination will not be necessary, inspection of the eyes is still applicable.
2. The examiner must maintain composure and express confidence. It is extremely important to identify this patient's concerns and needs through active listening and therapeutic discussion. It is important to be as precise as possible and to set limits as appropriate.

Content Review Questions

Multiple Choice

1. a	9. b
2. c	10. a
3. b	11. d
4. d	12. c
5. a	13. a
6. d	14. b
7. c	15. d
8. c	

CHAPTER 25

Terminology Review

1. Primary amenorrhea
2. RED-S
3. Sports-related concussion
4. Atlantoaxial instability
5. Oligomenorrhea

Concepts Application

Preparticipation Component	Questions to be Asked/Data to be Included
Medical History	Past and present medical conditions Surgeries Medications and supplements Allergies
General Questions	Any issues you wish to discuss Any previous denial or restriction on sports participation Current/ongoing medical problems
Heart Health (Self and Family)	**Self** Ever fully or nearly passed out during or after exercise Any discomfort, pain, tightness or pressure in chest during exercise Does heart ever race, flutter or skip beats during exercise Has a doctor ever said you have heart problems Ever had a heart test such as an EKG or Echocardiogram Any light headedness or more shortness of breath than your friends during exercise Ever had a seizure **Family** Has any family member or relative died of a heart problem, unexplained drowning or car accident or other sudden, unexplained death before age 35 Any family member with a genetic heart problem? Anyone with an implanted pacemaker or defibrillator before age 35
Bone and Joint	Ever had a stress fracture or other injury to a bone, muscle, ligament, joint or tendon that caused a missed practice or a game Any bone, muscle, ligament, joint or tendon injury that bothers you
Medical Questions	Cough, wheeze, or difficulty breathing during or after exercise Missing organ: kidney, eye, testicle, spleen or other Groin or testicle pain, painful bulge or hernia in groin area Recurring or "come and go" skin rashes including herpes or MRSA Any concussion or head injury that caused confusion, prolonged headache, or memory problems Any numbness, tingling, weakness in arms and legs, unable to move arms and legs after being hit or falling Ever become ill when exercising in heat Any sickle cell trait or disease – self or family Any past or present eye or vision problems Any worry about your weight Trying to or recommended to lose or gain weight Any special diet or do you avoid certain food or food groups Ever had an eating disorder
Females only	Ever had a menstrual period Age at first menstrual period Date of most recent menstrual period Number of periods in last 12 months

Clinical Reasoning

1. a. Stage 1 Hypertension
   b. Two additional blood pressure measurements should be obtained in the subsequent weeks. If his blood pressure is consistently elevated, an evaluation should be conducted for an etiology and for end-organ damage.
   c. Assess for use of substances known to increase blood pressure such as over-the-counter supplements, alcohol, tobacco, and highly caffeinated beverages.
   d. Contact

2. a. Complex
   b. Neuropsychological testing and consultation with a multidisciplinary team that includes a sports medicine physician with experience in concussion management

Content Review Questions

Multiple Choice

1.	b	9.	c
2.	c	10.	c
3.	a	11.	a
4.	d	12.	b
5.	a	13.	c
6.	b	14.	a
7.	d	15.	b
8.	b		

CHAPTER 26

Terminology Review

1. Penetrating trauma
2. Hypoxemia
3. Upper airway obstruction
4. Shock state
5. Ventilatory failure
6. Secondary assessment
7. Durable power of attorney
8. Blunt trauma
9. Status asthmaticus
10. Primary assessment
11. Increased intracranial pressure
12. Pulmonary embolism
13. Advance directive
14. Status epilepticus
15. ABCs

Application to Clinical Practice

Concepts Application

1. Primary
2. Primary
3. Secondary
4. Primary
5. Secondary
6. Secondary
7. Primary
8. Primary
9. Secondary
10. Primary

Case Study

1. Findings:
   A. Has open airway; is moving air and is able to speak
   B. Respiratory distress; dyspnea with nasal flaring
   C. Circulation—has some cyanosis around lips; should palpate pulses
2. Administration of oxygen
3. Vital signs

4. Data deviating from normal: The respiratory data, dyspnea with bloody sputum, and blood gas findings. His neurologic and mental status suggests hypoxia. Significant fact is that he had knee surgery 2 weeks ago.
5. The most serious concern to continue to monitor for (and treat) is the respiratory status. A priority would be to manage the airway and provide ventilatory assistance because the laboratory findings indicate he does not have adequate ventilation. Chest radiography would be helpful.
6. This young man is in serious trouble, and if the respiratory status does not improve, death may follow. Initial data suggest an acute pulmonary embolus. Another problem to rule out is drug overdose.

Completion

1.
   A Alert: no stimuli needed
   V Verbal stimuli: responsive to
   P Painful stimuli: responsive to
   U Unresponsive to verbal and pain stimuli
2.
   A Allergies
   M Medications or drugs of any type currently being taken by the patient
   P Past illnesses (e.g., diabetes, epilepsy, hypertension); Pregnancy
   L Last meal
   E Events preceding the precipitating event; Environment related to the injury

Clinical Reasoning

1. a. Burns and being in a house fire should immediately alert any healthcare provider to the possibility of smoke, heat, and chemical inhalation. Injuries to the respiratory system may be the most significant injury that these patients sustain.
   b. Young children and infants have small nasal and oral airway passages; shorter, narrower tracheas; and shorter necks. The larynx is higher and more anterior as well. These differences affect airway management. Children also have a large body surface area. Children who have sustained burns to the skin are more susceptible to fluid losses, hypothermia, and infection than are adults.

Content Review Questions

Multiple Choice

1.	a	9.	c
2.	c	10.	c
3.	b	11.	d
4.	c	12.	d
5.	a	13.	b
6.	d	14.	c
7.	d	15.	a
8.	a		